HEALTH POLICY AND REFORMS

HEALTH POLICY AND REFORMS

Governance in Primary Healthcare

Council for Social Development

K. B. Saxena

HEALTH POLICY AND REFORMS
Governance in Primary Healthcare
K. B. Saxena

First Published, 2010

ISBN 978-93-5002-049-4 (Pb)

Published by
AAKAR BOOKS
28 E Pocket IV, Mayur Vihar Phase I, Delhi-110 091
Phone : 011-2279 5505 Telefax : 011-2279 5641
aakarbooks@gmail.com; www.aakarbooks.com

Printed at
Arpit Printographers, Delhi-110 032
arpitprinto@yahoo.com

Contents

Preface

The development discourse, in recent times, has been replete with the words/terms introduced by the international agencies which replace their traditional meanings and redefine them to conform to their ideological needs. 'Governance' is one such word in this vocabulary introduced by the World Bank to assess whether development projects have achieved their declared objectives. It has conceptualized governance in a manner that shifts focus from policy to implementation, signifying thereby that the policies are beyond contest. Only the process of translating these policies into desired outcomes is material to its success. Governance is viewed in this framework as a technocratic exercise which can deliver the results expected of them, if properly designed structures of decision making are in place and autonomy of decision making is provided to them.

This paper does not share this construct of governance and its implicit dichotomy between policy and implementation. Governance can neither be delinked from policy and its deeply conflictive dimensions, nor can the delivery system operate in a sanitized environment unaffected by tensions generated by the unequal social structure and manipulative power of the dominant interests. The outcome of governance autonomous of these considerations would lead to inequitious outcomes and exacerbate social conflict.

Governance as conceptualized in the Tenth Five-Year Plan is more broad based so as to include social sensitivity, transparency, equity, accountability, participation and absence of discrimination. Taking this normative frame, governance issues with reference to the various facets of the public health system in the rural areas have been discussed. As the neo-liberal transformation of economy has impacted on the health policy, the imprint of this change on the public health system has also been dealt with. Admittedly, the treatment of issues is very brief and does not purport to have covered all their major dimensions. It was also not possible to do so within the scope of a paper since a lot of literature exists on each facet of public health covered here. The discussion on issues has also been followed by an analysis of the interests impinging on health governance. The last section attempts to explore a suitable conceptual frame to position health governance issues with reference to the two paradigms which have sought to explain the happenings in the organization of medicine.

The paper was written in 2006 for the project 'Public Report on Health', which the Council for Social Development is implementing. The original plan of the project authority to publish all the background papers it had commissioned was given up due to certain unavoidable constraints. Meanwhile, the Government introduced the National Rural Health Mission in 2005 as a major policy intervention to address most of the issues raised in this paper. Its operations started in 2006. This required major changes incorporating measures taken in respect of each facet of public health touched upon here and commending on whether they would resolve the problems raised therein. It has, however, not been possible to do so considering the amount of work involved as also the need to give sufficient time for these measures to be implemented before commenting on their impact. But the paper has included a section on the Mission activities and some comments based on the first year's performance. By now, the second year's performance has been evaluated and the third year's evaluation is in the pipeline. The Mission has, therefore, generated considerable information on the overall and state-wise performance which would require a separate paper to deal with even briefly. It is proposed to undertake this exercise after the Mission has completed its five-year tenure in 2010.

While writing this paper, I have drawn upon the institutional resources of the Council for Social Development which is acknowledged with gratitude. I also thank Aakar Books who have taken great interest in publishing it.

K.B. Saxena

Chapter 1

Concerns of Governance in Health Sector

Governance, in the conventional sense, signifies actions of the government to rule according to norms (Brass, 2002). This essentially implies decision making to set political goals, determining strategies to realize them, identifying agencies and structures for delivery and monitoring the outcomes for making corrective interventions, where necessary. Against the backdrop of neo-liberal ascendancy of the global economy, the World Bank has transformed the meaning of governance to imply measures to replace the state with non-state agencies as instruments for implementation of decisions and to facilitate the operation of market economy. This change focused on the dimension of governance relating to implementation, taking the goal setting or policy making as settled, which political leaders cannot alter (Mohanty, 2007). Globalization has created a conundrum in this discourse (Ludden, 2005). It has shifted the policy setting to diverse actors across the world with different interests, priorities and commitments. National governments are left with no power to determine goals they must promote but, on the other hand, are saddled with the responsibility to deliver outcomes of the policy settled externally. They are, therefore, unable to govern development. In the changed discourse, governance is increasingly viewed as a technocratic exercise which can be carried out by acting according to rationally laid-down norms. The agencies can be trusted to deliver if the structures of decision making are put in place and autonomy is provided to them. This construct of governance as an apolitical phenomenon is seriously flawed. Neither can governance be delinked from policy and its deeply conflicting dimensions nor can the delivery system operate in a sanitized environment unaffected by tensions generated as a result of the unequal social structure and manipulative power of its dominant interests. The outcome of governance in such a frame would produce highly iniquitous outcomes and exacerbate conflicts. The health sector in India is an example par excellence of this conflict in the current discourse on governance.

Development is among the core functions of any government since it is perceived as something good and desirable. Governing development relates to the process of translating development goals into deliverable benefits for producing the desired outcomes. The notion of development is conditioned by the conceptual frame of national economy which can be considered to have passed through three distinct phases since Independence. The period up to the mid-1980s constitutes, broadly, the first phase characterized by a 'welfare-centric' approach. From the beginning of the second phase in the mid-1980s, a distinct shift is discernable in the macro-economic management towards market orientation with a focused and forceful thrust emerging from the acceptance of Structural Adjustment Programme in the early 1990s. The period since 1995, making up the third phase, has seen the development paradigm distinctly moving towards a progressive integration with the global regime of investment, finance and trade, further intensifying its neo-liberal underpinnings and anchoring policy making to global institutions and processes. The three phases broadly coincide with a similar evolution of the international economy since the Second World War. Development policies, irrespective of the sector involved, essentially bear the imprint of these economic changes since they involve distribution and utilization of resources generated by the economy. The health sector is an important component of development since the health status of the population determines the productivity of economy and well being of the nation. Governance issues in the health sector emerge from the processes of setting policy goals, laying down strategies, instruments and structures for rendering them into tangible services and the social environment impinging on decision making in this regard. These issues essentially centre on the distribution of healthcare facilities, entitlements of people seeking health intervention, accessibility to services, quality of care received and space available to them to influence these decisions.

In the Indian context, concerns of governance in the health sector arise from four factors. The first relates to the low level of health indices in human development in India compared with the other developing countries of the same category. These are mirrored in the high IMR and MMR rates,[1] faltering immunization coverage,[2] stagnating nutritional status of children, unrelenting levels of mortality from communicable diseases (TB[3] and Malaria,[4] HIV-AIDS,[5] Diarrhoea[6]), increasing number of deaths from non-communicable diseases (cancer, CVD, diabetes), huge number of persons suffering from various forms of disabilities—visual, hearing, locomotive and mental—and very high levels of nutritional deficiencies in all age groups. This is despite an investment of Rs. 126.27 billion (1998) in health services and a huge infrastructure—145,272 sub-centres, 22,370 primary health centres, 4,045 community health centres[7] , 550 district hospitals and the number of beds estimated at 95,000 (taking into account the private sector which provides the bulk of curative healthcare services). The human resources available consist of 523,000 allopathic doctors and 11,5000 practitioners of other systems and 566,000 nursing staff.

The second is that a very large section of the population (those belonging to BPL) has no access/reliable access to healthcare despite a fair spread of primary healthcare infrastructure. They either do not seek medical care due to cost consideration or access the most unqualified practitioners who practise in violation of the law. This could imply that either very little of the health budget is spent on the poor or the resources do not reach the frontline service providers or the motivation for delivery of services is weak or there is a lack of demand from the poor (Devrayan and Shah, 2004). Alternatively, they are either inaccessible or prohibilitively expressive in dysfunctional and unresponsive to the needs of the people (World Bank, 2004).

The third is reflected in a very low level of utilization of rural public health services paradoxically existing along with the first and the second. The fourth emerges from the wide geographical and regional disparities in distribution and quality of healthcare services and social inequalities in access to them which have impact on their utilization and health outcomes.

Chapter 2

Governance in Rural Healthcare: Pre-Reform Period

Of the three segments of the health system—public, private and voluntary—this paper is essentially focused on the public health sector where the government is directly involved. Even in the segment of the public health system, this paper is confined to rural healthcare for a variety of reasons. The rural areas have the largest presence of public healthcare institutions. Rural healthcare is, therefore, institutionally and predominantly public. The majority of population still resides in the rural areas and, therefore, its access to healthcare decisively influences the health outcomes of the people in the country. The structure and range of health services in the rural areas are significantly different from those in the urban areas. The healthcare services in rural areas is a post-Independence development and has faced challenges from their inception. This system consists of a pyramid type of structure at whose bottom is the sub-centre which moves up to the second tier called the Primary Health Centre, thereafter to the third tier known as Community Health Centre. The fourth tier is designated as the District Hospital and at the top of the structure is the medical college hospital. The bottom three tiers are known as the Primary Health Care, the facilities at the district (also the sub-district) level are labeled as secondary healthcare and the teaching hospitals are considered to be the tertiary care facilities. The different tiers have been conceived with inbuilt linkages to provide the needed services. The medical college hospitals are largely located in the towns and usually constitute a part of the urban healthcare in view of the structure of their organization and the range of services they provide.

The Tenth Five-Year Plan [Vol. 1, Chapter 6), conceptualized features of good governance, irrespective of the sectoral context, as the 'exercise of legitimate political power, and formulation and implementation of policies and programmes that are equitious, transparent, non-discriminatory, socially sensitive, participatory, and above all, accountable to the people at large. There could, however, be aspects of governance that are contextually driven and geared to address the local concerns' [Planning Commission, 2002]. Taking this normative frame, the governance issues can be discussed with reference to the various facets of the public health system in the rural areas which, in their totality, present problems to citizens seeking health intervention face while accessing services provided therein. These revolve round the following: (a) Policy parameters, (b) Availability (distribution of infrastructure and services), (c) Instrumentality (mode of provisioning), (d) Functionality (operational arrangements which lend effectiveness to the availability of services), (e) Access (conditions which ensure that services would be available when sought), (f) Quality (level of care which provides reasonable satisfaction), (g) Management—internal (ability to tie up various inputs in healthcare delivery), Management—external: social determinants (inter-sectoral synergies to promote good health), (h) Equity (which makes access to healthcare non-discriminatory and socially sensitive), and (i) Social control (which make healthcare participatory and accountable).

The governance issues in rural healthcare can be discussed in respect of these facets with reference to the dimensions indicated against each as per the following chart:

(*a*) Policy Parameters

(*b*) Instrumentality { Provider agency
Financing

(*c*) Availability { Norm and location
Geographical spread
Range of services

Internal constraints-human resources, infrastructure and supplies

(*d*) Functionality	External constraints: referral system, health information, disease surveillance
(*e*) Accessibility	Geographical barriers Social barriers Income barriers Gender barriers Disability and Age barriers
(*f*) Quality	Public: Standards, Monitoring Private: Regulation
(*g*) Equity	
(*h*) Management (internal)	Organizational: Ministry (Central) Departments (States) Health planning Programme structures, Medicinal systems Inputs—Drugs, supplies, HRM procurement and maintenance Medical education Health systems research
Management (external)	Inter-sectoral: Social determinants
(i) Social Control	Community participation Decentralization, Health Education Accountability

Policy

Health policy goals have followed the imperatives of the national economy and reflect changes in tandem with its thrust. Of the three phases in the evolution of the economy, the public health sector was central to the provision of services as well as promoting social determinants of health in the first phase. The private sector began to be promoted as an alternative provider of curative health services in the second phase since the mid-1980s and eventually emerged as the dominant provider in the subsequent phase. The public health sector in the later two phases was confined largely to preventive and promotive care, disease control programmes and emergency services. The facilities in the first phase were mostly in the public health sector and, therefore, limited in availability but more equitably distributed and undifferentiated in access. Healthcare became diversified in the mode of provisioning and its units increased in number but were skewed in spread and differentiated in access and quality of care in the second phase. This trend is getting reinforced in the third phase. The coverage was universalistic in the first phase. There was no stipulation of any payment and therefore the services could be accessed by any needy person. The range of services provided was also not restricted though quality content was limited. They were curtailed to segmented care and became restricted in coverage and differentiated in entitlements depending upon one's capacity to pay in the subsequent phases. The primacy of market, progressive withdrawal of the state in provisioning of healthcare and commodification of healthcare supply became the hallmark of health policy transformation in the second and the third phases, which impacted on the quality of care in the public health system as well. With the onset of globalization, healthcare has virtually shed its 'service' character and emerged as a global commodity. Community participation, an integral part of the health policy in the first phase, was conceived as an instrument of subjecting health services to a modicum of social accountability. This has given way to consumer choice in the second phase consistent with market-centric healthcare. The third phase has increasingly witnessed erosion of social accountability and its virtual replacement by accountability to the international institutions and interests. These changes had their impact on the management of the public health system. It faced pressures to accommodate the market-driven changes and imperatives of globalization.

Social Environment

The social environment impinging on health governance also reflects a distinct transformation. The first dimension of this change relates to the role of democratic institutions. In the first phase, political leaders and institutions were active players in designing health policy, influencing processes of delivery and holding Government accountable. This could be observed in the pressures exerted on the Government for provision of healthcare facilities in the underserved areas, lobbying for setting up of healthcare institutions in their states/ constituencies, expansion of and improvement in services provided by the existing healthcare institutions, making complaints about non-availability of health personnel and essential drugs, pleading for equitable spread of medical education facilities, and investigating infrastructure and intervention to control drug prices. There was little restraint on this active role by way of pressure exerted by the private sector except in the manufacturing and pricing of drugs where the multinational drug industry had a dominating presence.

In the second phase, a distinct de-politicization of health governance was observed. The decisions on all these and other issues of health policy and operative aspects began to be taken not on the basis of assessment derived from the feedback gathered through political processes but purely on economic rationality delinked from social and political ramifications. Excessive importance was given to the financial and technical aspects of programme selection and, therefore, to the technocratic advice. The political institutions and processes as instruments of distributive healthcare and enforcing accountability of providers became irrelevant. The World Bank-funded programmes were classic examples of this undemocratic nature of governance since a distrust of politics in decision making was embedded in the structure of their management. This had implications for the accountability and effectiveness of health services and the capacity and autonomy of decision making. The third phase has relegated decisions on these issues to the institutions and interests outside the nation state and, therefore, seriously jeopardized the national accountability for outcomes that emerge from these decisions.

The second dimension of social environment is signified by barriers in access to healthcare. The first phase in this regard was dominated by inequalities in social structure driven by considerations of caste, class, ethnicity, gender and disability, which generated differentiated access to healthcare services and the quality of care received notwithstanding the preponderance of the public health system in provision of healthcare and universal nature of entitlements. The groups affected by these barriers faced discrimination from providers or were constrained to use these services optimally for other reasons. These barriers, far from getting reduced with large-scale provisioning of healthcare in the private sector in the second and third phases, exacerbated further. The income differentials and cost of care prevented these marginalized groups from seeking access to private healthcare because it was unaffordable. When confronted with serious illness, they were forced to access unqualified providers. The excessive patient load, introduction of user charges, outsourcing of some services to private agencies, etc. also constrained their access to public healthcare, particularly the OPD.

Instrumentality

Instrumentality refers to the modes/institutions/agencies through which healthcare is delivered and the manner of financing expenditure relating to it. These modes can be of three types: public, private for profit, private without profit/ charitable/non-governmental. The public agencies are institutions established by the Government where the expenditure incurred for delivering healthcare is met from public resources, the bulk of which comes from tax collection. The health seeker gets services from such institutions free of cost. Usually, these services are available to all without any discrimination and levy of fee from patients who access them. The private for profit mode refers to healthcare institutions which are managed by individual professionals, entrepreneurs or corporate agencies with their own resources or capital borrowed from the financial institutions. The services are not free here and the health seeker has to pay for availing of them. For this reason, the access is limited to those who have the ability to pay. The organizations belonging to the third category are those which, by and large, provide healthcare services free of cost or at a nominal/subsidized cost and whose entire or major portion of expenditure is met by some charitable institutions or periodic grant received from the Government.

Provider Agency

In the pre-colonial period of India, institutional forms of delivery of health services in the current sense of the term did not exist. Individuals were not formally trained but acquired knowledge of medicine/healing through traditional modes of learning. They inherited these skills as professional acquisition from the family as the practice of medicine was usually a caste-based occupation. Sporadic institutional health services did exist in some towns or centres of pilgrimage. Such institutions delivered healthcare services to patients free and were financed by rulers or through charities. During the colonial period, hospitals/dispensaries were set up and financed by the Government. But their spread was confined mostly to urban centres which were enclaves of the British civil administration and cantonments. These healthcare units catered to patients from the ruling class. The private sector healthcare, as a distinct and fairly large (more than 70%) segment of services emerged in the form of private practitioners both in the system of Western medicine as well as traditional medicine. The private practitioners obviously charged fees and, therefore, could be accessed only by those who had the necessary resources to meet this cost. After Independence, based on the Bhore Committee Report, the responsibility to provide preventive, promotive and curative health services was entrusted to the Government. The expenditure over it was to be met from public funds and healthcare services were admissible to all without discrimination and irrespective of the capacity to pay. The rural-urban disparities in availability of healthcare were sought to be bridged by establishing healthcare units with an equitable spread in the rural areas. The Government constituted the instrument of delivery as well as provided the finances for healthcare services. National Health Policy (1983) (MoHFW, 1983)—the first such formal declaration, while reiterating the commitment to universal and comprehensive primary healthcare, introduced a caveat for the first time that these services would be provided at a cost which people can afford implying that healthcare services would not be entirely free. It also incorporated the thinking that the private sector should also be involved in the provision of curative services in view of the 'constraint of resources' with the Government and advocated encouragement of private investment in the sector. This indicated a distinct shift in the health policy process towards privatization of healthcare services. The impact of this change could be observed in rapid expansion of private sector healthcare with state subsidies and concessional finance. The model of healthcare adopted by the Government in the post-1990s, has curtailed the 'comprehensive' primary healthcare to 'selective' primary healthcare, which narrows down the ambit of primary healthcare to reproductive and child health, immunization, control of selective diseases and emergency services. For the remaining health problems, the health seeker has to access private healthcare services. Public hospitals do exist and are available to all those interested in availing of their services but are constrained by resources and have introduced a filtering process by way of user charges for some services to meet this deficit. These changes have led to a phenomenal growth of private healthcare segment which has now become the dominant mode in provision of curative healthcare services. The public investment in health has declined and public healthcare institutions suffer from poor infrastructure, neglected maintenance, shortage of personnel and financial resources with acute pressure of the patients which affect access to them and quality of care they provide. The expansion of infrastructure to meet the increasing patient load has also virtually stopped. This thrust in policy is the direct outcome of the changed political economy which requires reduced state involvement in provision of social services. The result is curtailment in expenditure on programmes in the social sector of which health is a major sub-sector. This has affected access to healthcare services of a large number of people who cannot afford to meet its cost. The inability to avail of healthcare has negative implications for the health status of such people and, therefore, of the country. The private-without-profit health sector is too small to have any impact on the overall position. Its expansion is severely constrained by the lack of sustainable resources, whether from philanthropists or the Government. Since access to and quality healthcare has a decisive impact on the health status of the people, the choice of the mode of provisioning healthcare which can ensure this access to all, particularly the poorer sections, and render quality healthcare emerges as a serious governance issue.

Financing of expenditure

The mode of financing healthcare directly determines the nature of provider agency and affordability of access. The healthcare financed with public expenditure translates into equitable distribution of health facilities, universalization of access, greater pressure for quality of care and more efficient utilization of resources all of which affect the health outcomes. In the period prior to the 1990s, particularly from the fifth to seventh Plan period, major investments were made in rural healthcare via the Minimum Needs Programme which showed considerable improvements in the health status of the population. This trend was reversed following the Structural Adjustment Programme with the onset of the 1990s when resource commitments to the public health sector were reduced. The curtailment of public expenditure in the health sector incapacitated the public health sector with shortage of personnel, neglected maintenance, non-functional equipments, inadequate consumables, non-availability of drugs and affected the quality of care which was acknowledged as such in the National Health Policy (2002) (MoHFW, 2002[a]). This was accompanied by privatization measures such as introduction of user charges from patients, outsourcing of services to private agencies, restricting the range of services to be provided. The two had the effect of substantially increasing out-of-pocket spending on health with debilitating effects which were observed in increasing avoidance to seek healthcare,[8] indebtedness, and deteriorating economic conditions. India accounts for one of the highest total health expenditures among countries of comparable status but more than 80% of it is out of pocket. A meagre 5% of households have obtained some kind of insurance cover for at least one member (JSA, 2009). It has one of the lowest public expenditures on health (0.9% of the GDP and 18.22% of the total expenditure on health till recently). This has manifested in poor health outcomes despite the fast rate of economic growth. The priority issue of governance is to radically alter the iniquitous financing pattern by substantially increasing public investments in health. But it is also about achieving allocative efficiencies in public health expenditure. The allocative inefficiencies are reflected in the inter-programme distribution of resources not dictated by objective norms, insufficient allocation for operational expenses of healthcare compared to the salaries component, rural-urban disparities in provisioning of services, etc. The mode of financing should also have the focused objective to provide protection to the poorer sections from the high cost of healthcare, particularly catastrophic illness/episodes and easy and universal access to quality healthcare.

Availability of health services

Norm and Location

Since the rural areas at the time of Independence were extremely deficient in health infrastructure, setting up primary healthcare institutions consisting of three tiers, i.e. Sub Centres, Primary Health Centres and Community Health Centres as per the Bhore Committee Reports assumed top priority. This infrastructure was to be established on the basis of norms specifying the unit of population each tier was expected to serve (Sub-centre for a population of 5000, Primary Health Centre for a population of 30,000 and Community Health Centre to serve the needs of 1,20,000 population). These norms were relaxed in the case of hilly, inaccessible and tribal areas (3000 for sub-centre, 20,000 for Primary Health Centre and 80,000 for Community Health Centre). This task could not be fully accomplished due to several reasons—resource constraints, slow pace of construction, remoteness of areas and absence of political clout from difficult areas to exert requisite pressure, etc. The implementation process was also marked by politically-driven distortions in the location and distribution of these centres. The predominately tribal areas, hilly areas and sparsely populated geographical areas remained under-provided, while the developed regions and constituencies of influential political leaders were better covered. This skewness in the distribution of facilities was not levelled even by locating health facilities relating to the non-allopathic (ISM and Homoeopathy) streams. Good governance lay in prioritizing transfer of resources towards these neglected areas inhabited by the marginalized social groups for setting up health centres and deployment of health personnel against competing demands from powerful social groups and accelerating pace of construction work. This did not happen. With the shift in health policy, state commitment to expansion of health infrastructure took a back seat and other mechanisms of financing it (private sector, NGO, etc.) began to be explored and encouraged. The Tenth Five-Year Plan restricted setting up of new primary healthcare institutions or their construction only to the exceptionally difficult areas where the private sector is unwilling to establish its presence. This implies that the norm-based supply of healthcare facilities to keep up with the increasing demand is virtually being abandoned. This can be seen in the progress of growth of infrastructure in the public health sector in the rural areas which has shown a sharp decline between 2002 and 2007. The increase in the number of Sub Centres is less than 6%. The strength of PHCs has gone down by more than 2%. Only CHCs have registered an increase. The achievement in creation of new infrastructure in the Tenth Five-Year Plan is 76% in the case of Sub Centres, 13% for PHCs and 37% for CHCs of the targets set therein (JSA, 2009), which is considerably lower.

The deficiency in availability of health infrastructure in the underserved areas cannot be met by the private sector or NGOs. The former would have no interest in establishing such facilities because of its non-viability in terms of returns from fees charged for services. The NGOs are dependent upon funding either by the Government or charitable agencies and therefore have no financial capacity of their own to set up such arrangements. Though the private sector is fast expanding and has already emerged as a dominant provider, its infrastructure is even more skewedly distributed. The expansion has largely concentrated in urban and prosperous rural areas where people have higher purchasing power. No degree of encouragement and concessions have persuaded them to move to the underserved areas. The skewness in availability of health facilities has been a feature not only between the regions of a state but across states as well. The states endowed with better resource position are able to provide more extensive health infrastructure to service their population while the poorer states continue to lag behind. The federal mechanisms for resource transfer to the states have not neutralized this inequality. Thus, making a minimum level of health services available to the people in areas neglected by the development process continues to be a major governance issue. The resolution of this problem would directly influence the reduction in adverse health indices, such as rates of infant and maternal mortality, neonatal, antenatal and postnatal mortality and reduction in total fertility rate and morbidity levels in the affected areas.

The National Rural Health Mission (MoHFW, 2005) has promised to address this concern. The problem of non-availability of health services in tribal and hilly areas is sought to be tackled through provision of mobile medical services from a nearby fully functional health facility which may cover different villages periodically. Even such arrangements, symbolic as they are, have floundered because of non-availability of assured transport, high cost of mobility, inadequate coverage, irregular visits, lack of cooperation from health service providers and absence of monitoring their effectiveness.

Geographical spread

Geographical disparities are reflected in the rural-urban differentials in availability of healthcare facilities in terms of hospitals, beds as well as quality of services (Jessani and Anantharaman, 1993; Kethineni, 1991). The rural areas have 15 times lower number of hospital beds and six times lesser number of doctors. The skewness in per capita fund allocation for health between the rural and urban areas is 1:7. The non-functionality of primary healthcare facilities and poor quality of services rendered in the rural areas has pushed people to seek healthcare in better equipped urban hospitals. In terms of public health sector financing, the distribution of resources is skewed between the rural and urban areas with over 60% of allocations going to the latter where only 40% of the population resides. On a per-capita basis, the rural areas get only half of what is available to the urban areas and, of this, a negligible percentage goes towards curative care and capital expenditure. The public health spending is 70% in urban areas and only 30% in rural areas (Duggal, 2005). The urban bias in resource allocation for health is very sharply reflected in the level of curative care available and its quality. This rural-urban differential is not confined to the allopathic medicine but also extends to the ISM and Homoeopathy streams which is reflected in the number of their facilities, doctors and beds in the two areas. In the post-reform period, this rural-urban divide has widened further. The expansion of curative care facilities in the private sector is concentrated in the urban areas or prosperous rural pockets, which reinforces the existing disparities. The geographical disparities, which also include imbalances between different areas within the states reflecting the uneven pattern of development, have been a recurrent theme in the discourse on health. The recently launched National Rural Health Mission is committed to improving the functionality of rural health services but does not target addressing the geographical disparities in any focused and substantial manner.

Range of Facilities

The availability of health services is also judged by the range of services provided in the healthcare units in relation to the needs of the population. The primary healthcare infrastructure is poorly equipped in this regard. There is no provision for attending to the health problems arising out of a degraded environment resulting from development activities—industrialization, urbanization, intensive agriculture and infrastructural expansion. These problems are caused by pollution of air quality, water sources and degradation of land

and biodiversity, which have also affected livelihood of people and their productivity. The healthcare units have no infrastructure and health personnel to deal with the serious ailments caused by these factors. Further, due to the poor regulatory norms regarding industrial hazards and extremely lax enforcement of the existing norms, a host of occupational diseases has spread among the workers engaged in industrial units and people living in the vicinity. This danger is increasing with the relocation of many hazardous industries including those dealing with radioactive material from the West. But we have a negligible public health infrastructure to deal with occupational health which suffers from lack of attention and resources. The affected population, therefore, goes without even rudimentary care. This is compounded by virtually no action in waste management, particularly of the toxic variety, which contaminates the immediate environment. Even the Bhopal gas disaster has failed to prioritize this need in primary healthcare.

The increasing instances of suicides, depression, anxiety disorder also underline the need for availability of mental healthcare facilities in primary health care. More than a crore people need treatment for serious mental disorders while the incidence of mental illness affects 15 crore persons. Still, the country has no scheme, no resource allocation and no infrastructure relating to mental health built into the primary healthcare to undertake preventive, promotive and curative work. The meagre mental health programme currently under operation partially reaches out to 90 out of 600 districts. Even the requisite number of trained personnel for this discipline are not available (*Hindu*, 2009). With the demographic transition taking place, the country is aging fast. But geriatric medicine does not figure in the existing primary and secondary healthcare facilities.

These deficiencies in the range of services available in the primary healthcare deprive a large population from seeking health intervention. The NHRM has also omitted to provide these services in the revamped primary healthcare.

Functionality

The rural healthcare facilities are sub-optimally utilized. The level of utilization is determined by the functionality of these units which is affected by many problems. These problems can be broadly categorized into the constraints internal to the health unit and external constraints. The internal constraints include irrational distribution of facilities, deficient human resources, non-availability of drugs, non-functional equipments, inadequate contingency fund and poor infrastructure and maintenance. The external constraints relate to lack of requisite support for effective functioning, such as referral facilities, transport infrastructure, supplies, maintenance and finance, information collection and disease surveillance. These components of external inputs constitute the 'support system' which significantly contributes to the optimal utilization of facilities. In fact, the internal and external constraints are interrelated. The deficiencies which are internal to the facilities are relatable to the poor functioning of (external) support system. The most important components of this support system are referral and transport, without which the public health facilities at various levels cannot be linked.

Internal Constraints

The internal functionality of health units faces enormous problems. The Sub Centres are unevenly distributed. The population serviced by them is larger than the specified norm and, therefore, exceeds their capacity to handle it. They also suffer from irrational location defined by distance from the central area of habitation, lack of connectivity and transport problems as well as inadequate infrastructure support. These health units are also confronted with a shortfall in the strength of medical staff—ANMs 12.6% and Male Health Workers 53.4%. Of the functioning Sub Centres, 4711 are without the services of both ANMs and Male Health Workers. Even the staff available suffers from low level of workforce skills and motivation and ill-defined work profile (PHRN, 2006). The Sub Centres do not have essential drugs (iron-folic acid tablets, ORS packets and vitamin A syrup, vaccines for immunization which are contained in the drug kits) and instruments for antenatal and neonatal checkups. The PHCs face continuing criticism regarding non-availability of doctors (807 of them have no doctors) and paramedics (shortage of 41.1% of lab technicians and 17.1% of pharmacists (JSA, 2009), low OPD attendance and unutilized beds which leads to under-utilized manpower. The sub-optimal use of manpower is due to the poor infrastructure and facilities, paucity of skills, confidence and motivation in healthcare providers, absence of standard treatment guidelines, a non-functional referral system, non-availability of essential drugs, diagnostic facilities and equipments along with poor maintenance. The CHCs face serious constraints with regard to the gap in the sanctioned strength of specialists (nearly 65%) and paramedics, mismatch in deployment of personnel, infrastructural inadequacies relating to furniture, sanitation, drinking water, electricity, waste disposal, functional operation theatre, communication and transport, quality laboratory services besides non-availability of essential drugs, non-functional equipments, poor maintenance and insufficient contingency fund (PHRN, 2006). Of the functioning health units, 50% Sub Centres, 24% of PHCs and 16% CHCs are accommodated in rented or temporary premises. The knowledge and skill level of health personnel in these units is weak and their attitude towards service seekers harsh (JSA, 2009). The NRHM has brought in some improvement but it is inadequate.

The first level of support required is in respect of human resources, supplies, infrastructure, maintenance facilities and finances. The human resource support covers workforce management such as recruitment, deployment, training, motivation, skill updating, promotion and career progression of health providers. The infrastructure development and maintenance include renovation/construction of buildings, purchase, repair/replacement of equipments, provision of drinking water, electricity, sanitation and communication facilities. The supplies relate to procurement of equipments, drugs and consumables. The maintenance of equipments in working condition requires quick and timely attention to repairs, long-term contracts with suppliers and decisions about replacement. The drug procurement system involves preparation of a list of essential drugs, selection of drugs to be procured, timely placement of order, quality check, prompt distribution, budget planning and cost management. The financial management system essentially consists of mobilization of fund, timely distribution, its accounting and auditing. While some of these support systems do exist, they function inefficiently and aggravate governance problems. This is evident from the huge vacancies in the healthcare units at all levels of primary healthcare, mismatch in postings, absence of norm-based deployment and skewed distribution of personnel. The lack of repairs and maintenance in buildings, absence of staff residences, numerous problems relating to drinking water, sanitation and electricity and non-functional telephones speak poorly of the infrastructure and its maintenance. The non-availability of essential drugs is a perennial problem which is caused by delays and corruption in placing orders, mismatch between drugs needed and those supplied, purchase of drugs with insufficient time in their expiry date and irrational distribution arrangements. The non-functional equipments remaining without repair or replacement for substantial periods are due to delays in decisions on service contracts and procurement of new ones and failure to train the operating staff with necessary skills. These problems with regard to supplies, whether of drugs or equipments, are attributed to the absence of an efficient procurement and monitoring system. The financial management evaluations have shown delay in release of funds, failure to spend funds on the one hand and allocation of insufficient funds under some heads on the other, backlog in preparation and finalization of accounts and their audit leading to non-release of instalments from the Central government/donors and cash flow interruptions. All these issues have dominated the discourse on health governance.

EXTERNAL SUPPORT

Referral Arrangements

The effective functioning of primary healthcare rests on the principle that if a patient cannot be treated with the available facilities at the PHC, he/she should be immediately referred to the higher level health unit, i.e. the CHC. If the illness is beyond the capability of the CHC to handle, the patient should be referred to the District Hospital. The referral arrangements also imply that in serious cases, the lower unit should have facilities to transport the patient to the higher level health unit without delay to save life. The referral assistance is also required to access expert consultation and diagnostic services of the tertiary care institutions. These referral arrangements either do not exist in most places or are not functional and effective. The weak or non-existent referral system can also be caused by lack of connectivity between the PHC and CHC and CHCs and district hospital with a motorable road and a regular transport service. The result is that people prefer to access a higher level of health unit as the first choice to avoid risk to the patient's life. The inefficiency and ineffectiveness of referral arrangements has led to the under-utilization of the primary healthcare facilities and overload at the hospitals. The people tend to approach the hospitals even when the illness is not life threatening. This makes the hospital services cost ineffective and primary healthcare cost inefficient. The absence of referral support also makes health education programmes unattractive to the people. The inability of the Government to arrange effective referral systems with transport facilities has been a serious governance issue and has been widely commented upon in the discourse on the health system.

Health Information

The epidemiological database in the country is very weak (Qadeer, 1995). There is no regular system of collection of information on the incidence of disease and the cause of death except what comes out from the hospital records. Much of the information which forms the basis for health planning is either very old or has been derived from a small sample in research studies. This creates limitations in the understanding of disease, its history, social dimensions, changing incidence, geographical spread and the impact of environmental factors impinging on it. In this context, even the most elementary data collection system relating to death and birth registration suffers from weak organization, inadequate awareness, incapacity to mobilize existing institutional resources, insufficient financial commitment and low level of attention from policy-making establishment. The need for regular collection (periodical) of epidemiological information has been stressed by medical experts associated with health planning (Banerjee, 2005). National Health Policy, 2002 (MoHEW, 2002[a]) envisages completion of baseline estimates for the incidence of communicable diseases and to put in place statistical methods for updating these estimates to facilitate evidence-based policy making. The non-communicable diseases would have to wait longer for such an initiative. It also recognizes the need to establish National Health Accounts. There is little knowledge in the public domain about the progress made in this direction, which signifies the low priority given to this task.

Disease Surveillance

The other support required is with regard to the disease surveillance system which collects information on the profile of diseases and conveys it to the public health facilities to enable them to take timely technical and management decisions. This needs to be supplemented by research in public health which provides epidemiological analysis of diseases, their medical and social determinants.

The importance of effective disease surveillance for timely intervention when an epidemic breaks out or a major episode of illness strikes and its usefulness for health planning has been recognized by the Government. The absence of efforts to organize such an arrangement has figured as a serious governance issue. The subject resurfaces each time a major episode of illness occurs in a part of the country, infection spreads and unavoidable deaths take place due to the failure to take timely action. The critics have also stressed the need to involve local communities and panchayati raj institutions in this task. The absence of a rigorously laid-out drill to be followed for management of epidemics to limit the damage has also been observed. The ad hoc manner in which local administration intervenes without any prior preparedness even in areas where episodes of certain diseases occur periodically has exposed the acute incapacity of the local health agencies to undertake proper disease surveillance.

The existing disease surveillance system is weakly structured and suffers from lack of prioritization, paucity of human resource input, absence of efforts to seek people's participation and inability to achieve synergy between concerned institutions and programmes. It receives low attention in the overall planning and management of the public health system. The Government has taken up an externally funded project to institutionalize disease surveillance. While the attention this subject is now commanding is welcome, the health system governance should focus on more sustainable arrangements drawing upon the existing local resources—financial, man-power, institutional and non-official. As for the research input, the health system research is non-existent at the state level and below. Even its requirement is not considered essential by the state health policy establishment. It is viewed as an academic activity and, therefore, the exclusive preserve of the specialized central research institutions. The subject has not received adequate attention in the health system discourse.

The functionality of public health centres has been a major governance issue. The inadequacies and constraints in their functioning have figured in the official documents as well as public discourse. Good governance required that these deficiencies were addressed effectively. The problem of shortage of health personnel needed structural reforms in medical education. Human resource management reforms were necessary to tackle the myriad problems relating to recruitment, deployment, training, motivation, work ethic, behaviour of medical personnel and discipline and control over them. The maintenance of infrastructure required proper coordination with the concerned agencies of the Government. The constraints in availability of the physical infrastructure demanded that a dedicated organization be created exclusively for this purpose besides allocation of adequate resources to attend to the several problems connected with it in a holistic manner. The snags in supply of drugs and consumables could be addressed through a well thought-out procurement and distribution system and adequate financial provision. To avoid problems resulting from non-functional equipments, timely decisions on maintenance contract with suppliers and replacement were necessary. It is evident that sufficient and systematic action was not taken on these lines. With the change in political economy and health policy, the problems deteriorated on all fronts due to cutback in allocations, decision not to fill up vacant posts, restricted nature of care to be provided by public health units, reduced capital expenditure and brain drain to the private sector. The governance efforts, rather than addressing these issues for improving public health units, have shifted to encouraging the private health sector to take its place and become the dominant supplier of healthcare so that the pressure on public sector health units and, therefore, on government resources is reduced. In fact, the secondary and tertiary care services were asked even to generate their own resources by levying user charges for specific services. The cutback in public investment and distorted health personnel management led to an all-round deterioration in services. This forced the poor to access unqualified health providers or not to seek healthcare at all due to lack of resources and as a result, reduced the level of utilization of public health units. With better-off sections accessing private health care, there was no pressure on the Government to improve the functioning of public health units. The functionality of public health facilities thus emerges as a more serious governance issue at present than it was in the first phase. The NRHM has taken note of this crisis in the functionality of public healthcare and has included some measures to rejuvenate the system.

ACCESS

Barriers in availing of healthcare

Geographical

The access to health services is the key to realizing health policy goals. The availability of health facilities and their functional condition do contribute to the access of people to avail of services provided therein. This access is ab-initio constrained if the facilities are not available at a reasonable distance. This may happen either due to a lesser number of health units than the prescribed norm, which enlarges the jurisdiction of the existing units and the population to be served or uneven spatial distribution of available health units, which puts at a disadvantage the difficult areas for the same reason. The hilly, remote and tribal areas suffer from the latter constraint in access as they are underserved by these facilities. The functionality of the health units is another factor which constrains access. If the available facilities are not functional due to inadequacies mentioned earlier, it discourages the service seeker to access them. The hilly, tribal and remote areas also face non-functionality of the health units as a major problem due to the reluctance of the service providers to work there.

Location

But the access is not ensured even if the health facilities are available and are fully functional. The access to healthcare is constrained by several other factors, one of which relates to the location of the unit. The suitability of location is determined by its road connectivity and transport facilities, nearness to the centre of the economic activity or social life as well as the average distance covered by the population in its jurisdiction. The location decisions are often driven by political interests reflecting pulls and pressures from the competing groups. The unequal distribution of power among these groups impinges on the choice of location. These locational barriers vary from state to state and also within a state depending upon the level of development and the priority given to this work. The situation in Kerala is by far the best while large-sized states like MP, Bihar, UP, Jharkhand and Orissa present huge problems in this respect. The lack of political clout of the adversely affected population/ area is one factor in the failure to provide healthcare units as per norms and choose a rational location to ensure connectivity or reduce jurisdiction. The resource constraints have accentuated this barrier because setting up facilities, creating connectivity with an unsuitable location or reducing the size of jurisdiction have financial implications. The discourse on health governance has featured this issue.

Social

The social exclusion of SCs caused by caste, STs by ethnic and Muslims by communal bias affects their access to health services. This is evident from the disparity in respect of health indicators belonging to the population of these groups when compared to that of the general population. The SCs/STs have the most adverse profile in respect of IMR, under-5 Mortality Rate as well as the percentage of the malnourished. The STs fare even worse than the SCs in this respect. The Muslim minority has also low health indicators. This shows that the social biases operate at the level of service providers in public health facilities even when there is no discrimination in entitlements and the service is available free of cost. This phenomenon is widespread and can be observed in the delivery of other development programmes as well. There has been no intervention by the Government in terms of programme content, resource allocation, approach to delivery, training and orientation of service providers focused on this problem (Mishra et al., 2003).

Income

Income-based inequalities affect access to health services since a lot of expenditure has to be incurred on consultation and treatment. Those who do not have sufficient income are forced to ignore their health problems or take recourse to folk medicine/home-made remedies. This factor constrained access in the pre-reform period despite the universal coverage and free of cost entitlement in public health facilities. This is because some expenditure on availing of health services has to be incurred by the patient (such as cost of transport, drugs) even when public health facilities are accessed. Also, the poor can ill afford to lose a day's wage in accessing free care in a public health unit due to the time spent as it may be located at a considerable distance and overcrowded. These inequalities in access have increased with the growth of private sector healthcare, particularly in the post-reforms period. The access of the poor to the private sector health in-patient care, in any case, is less than the rich. The poor do seek private healthcare for out-patient services but this access is by and large from unqualified medical practitioners both for reasons of cost and the time saved. Overall, the poor, even though more vulnerable to disease, use both private and public health services less than the rich. At the primary care level, their participation is higher than at the secondary and tertiary levels because of the preventive programmes like immunization (Mishra et al., 2003). Bridging this gap in access, particularly to the public health services, has always been a challenge but has become more acute in the post-reforms period. The NRHM has sought to reduce this income by introducing a social health insurance scheme for in-patient care.

Gender

Gender-related barriers affect access of women (including children) to healthcare. These relate to the unsuitable timings of facilities, insensitivity of healthcare providers, absence of privacy in the clinics, indifference to their problems by the family, attitude of self-denial by women themselves and failure of the existing programmes to cover health problems experienced by women (Priya, 2001[b]). The constrained access of women to health services contributes to the adverse health outcomes for them. This can be observed in the high level of MMR and IMR, low percentage of institutional deliveries, very high percentage of nutritional deficiencies, high incidence of anaemia and increasing share of non-communicable diseases. The RCH (Reproductive and Child Health) and the earlier MCH (Maternal and Child Health) programmes have targeted some of these problems but with little appreciable success. The neglect of health problems of women other than those related to the reproductive aspects by these programmes is conditioned by the obsessive emphasis on family planning and has long been castigated in the public discourse on health both by experts as well as social activists [Qadeer, 2002; Sagar, 2001]. Despite the widespread critique of this approach, the resources and efforts invested in RCH programmes have failed to correct this distortion.

Disability and age

The ambit of primary healthcare has tended to ignore the special health problems of physically vulnerable groups who require special infrastructure and expertise in handling their healthcare. These are also the people who need healthcare most because of their own inability as also the incapacity of their family to look after their problems without expert assistance. These areas of health include occupational health, disability care, mental health, elderly care, interventions for social deviants. The lack of attention to these branches of medicine, more so in the context of the changing demographic profile and economic transition, is reflective of the inadequacy of health planning. The mainstreaming of these concerns in the existing structure of healthcare services and to promote specialized education and training for this purpose continues to be ignored even in the state health systems projects financed by the World Bank which envisage more comprehensive improvements in healthcare at the state level. The NRHM also does not incorporate any intervention in respect of this deficiency.

QUALITY OF CARE

Public Health System

The quality of healthcare is measured by two norms—the status of physical infrastructure and level of services provided. The quality of healthcare has all along figured as an issue of prime concern in the discourse on health governance. As long as the public-funded health system dominated the scene, the concern for quality in healthcare was subsumed under the more pressing issues relating to the supply of inputs to the facilities such as inadequate resource allocation for drugs, consumables and maintenance, absence of doctors and paramedics from duty and deficient infrastructure—physical (building, water supply, electricity) and investigative (functioning equipments). The under-utilization of primary healthcare was attributed to its poor quality on account of these deficiencies which determined its functional status. The quality of care is also signified by the level of satisfaction in treatment. The competence, approach and behaviour of doctors and other health personnel was not considered an important factor affecting the quality of services, whether rendered in the rural or urban healthcare. The declining degree of clinical supervision exercised by the higher level of medical personnel over the lower level of healthcare providers in the rural as well as the urban areas was, no doubt, recognized. But no measurable parameters were put in place for assessing the quality of medicare rendered in the public health system on this account. The issues relating to quality of care in terms of physical standards and service satisfaction have tended to emerge very sharply with the increasing commercialization of medicine, greater use of technology and enlarged presence of the private sector healthcare in the post-reforms period. The absence of consumer awareness on the one hand and a credible redressal mechanism to deal with the complaints of patients on the other helped to suppress cases of negligence and poor quality of treatment both in the rural and the urban healthcare in the pre-reforms period. These issues have begun to come up with increasing regularity and greater outburst of public anger in the urban areas both in public and private healthcare. The unethical practices of doctors in the public health system such as engaging in private practice and using their position in public health units to divert patients to their private clinics were widely known but not vigorously raised in the public domain in the absence of strong activist organizations in the civil society representing rights of the patients. This deficiency continues to exist. But the quality of healthcare is an even more serious issue in the private healthcare sector which has been discussed elsewhere in the paper. The quality of healthcare in both segments is integrally related to the regulation of healthcare which provides the standards for assessing it. This has remained a neglected issue in health governance though NHFS attempted to measure the quality of RCH programme in its 1998-99 survey (Mishra et al., 2003).

Standards

No attention was paid to laying down standards for promoting assurance of quality in the public health units. It was assumed that no such assurance was needed because of the 'public' nature of the facility, overall political accountability of health administration in the Government and the supervisory nature of control exercised by the higher level of formations within the public health organization. But the cases of negligence, neglect, insensitivity in treating patients in the public health facilities are enormous and often get reported in the media. Despite the 'public' nature of the facility, the failure to own mistakes and make amends for them has led, lately, to situations where the relations of victims have assaulted the medical staff on duty besides filing criminal cases against them. Thus, the public sector health facilities also need regulation by way of setting up standards for infrastructure and facilities as well as the level of services expected of them and a credible mechanism for grievance redressal. There has been little by way of any concrete action in this regard.

The NRHM, however, has made a small beginning in the matter. It has notified the Indian public health standards for a 24-hour PHC. This document provides the infrastructure, building plan, the equipment and drugs needed for a PHC to provide satisfactory nature of services. Similar Indian Public Health Standards have also been brought out in respect of a CHC. These standards also highlight the services these units are expected to provide. The standards for a Subcentre and a District Hospital on these lines are being worked out. But the Common Review Mission in its report has noted that 'often IPHS has been read only as a prescription of inputs, and not a prescription of outputs or as a service delivery guarantee. A focus on ensuring appropriate quantity and quality of service delivery outcomes to match any given level of inputs is not in place' (NRHM, 2007). The shortage of key personnel continues to adversely affect the delivery of services. The poor performance due to lack of accountability was also observed. Besides addressing the issue of filling vacant posts, periodic skill development training of health personnel, standard treatment protocols and regular monitoring are also required to enforce standards. On the behaviourial side, quality of interactions and information exchanges with patients and an attitude which does not convey impatience and intimidation is absolutely necessary. Health governance has to adequately capture these aspects in making requisite interventions. There is no indication that this is happening.

Monitoring

The assurance of quality is enforced through a dual mechanism of monitoring—internal and external. The internal mechanism consists of methods by which the health organization ensures that its guidelines of programmes are observed, standard treatment protocols adhered to and the quality is maintained in rendering services. This monitoring is carried out by maintenance of records, supervision, discussion on the information received and follow-up action. The performance in this regard is poor. The treatment protocols are not in place. The record maintenance suffers from lack of skills, guidance and training which is reflected in the quality of information collected and recorded. The rigour in data collection is lacking. The analysis of information and follow-up action on this basis is virtually non-existent. There is little by way of effective supervision in these matters although seniors do visit health units. Altogether, internal monitoring does not inspire confidence and, therefore, tells upon the quality of care.

The external mechanisms is an arrangement through which the stakeholders outside the health organization provide the feedback about the gaps in services, deficiencies in facilities and attitude and behaviour of service providers to create pressure on the delivery agencies to improve their performance. The external mechanism operates through the PRIs (Panchayati Raj Institutions), village health committees, patient welfare groups, elected representatives in state and central legislature, civil society organizations, media, etc. It functions as an instrument of enforcing social accountability of public health system and to create pressures for change and improvement in accordance with people's needs. The practice initiated under the NRHM to depute a team of experts and members of civil society to review the progress in respect of key parameters every year (called the Common Review Mission) is one such external mechanism.

Going by the findings of the Common Review Mission, November 2007, several gaps in the availability of services and quality of performance have been brought out which highlight the unresolved governance issues (NRHM, 2007).

The PRIs constitute an institutionalized and Constitutionally mandated external mechanism and are available nearest to the health seekers. This arrangement is democratic in character and independent of control of the public health organization and deserves to be effectively utilized for monitoring. The NRHM is committed to involve the PRIs and has set up the Village Health and Sanitation Committees and Rogi Kalyan Samitis for discharging this role. It also advocates utilization of NGOs in this task. But these structures are neither autonomous nor democratic. They are a creation of the health organization itself and are, therefore, ineffective in articulation of user interests and assertion with regard to the inadequacies in performance. They are also constrained by the nature of their composition, lack of clarity on the scope of their role and absence of capacity building for facilitation of their task. The PRIs, on the other hand, are constrained by inadequate authority and power and lack of knowledge and capacity to discharge their role.

Regulation

The urgency of introducing effective regulation of healthcare, particularly in the private sector, is currently the most discussed issue in health governance. In the early years of Independence, the need for regulation of healthcare was not acutely felt because the public sector healthcare had an edge in provision of services and was expected to be internally regulated through supervision. As the private sector began to increase its presence, encouraged by promotional efforts of the Government, the practices of private healthcare establishments came under scrutiny. The vulnerability of consumers to high cost, low level of care and risks to health and life from irrational medication, unnecessary investigations and negligence in treatment began to surface. The fragility of existing but inadequate and ineffective regulatory arrangements to check these features has been widely documented (Nandraj; 1994, Nandraj and Duggal, 1997). It also emerged that the institutions created for enforcement of standards and medical ethics miserably failed to discharge their responsibility both due to their structural weaknesses as also disinclination. The professional bodies have miserably failed to self regulate (Iyer and Jessani, 2000; Bhatt, 1996).

The public sector health services also failed to set standards and provide internal structures of self regulation and clinical protocols (Mishra et al., 2003). The strong consumer dissatisfaction with both sectors of healthcare led people to seek redressal under consumer protection law. The limitations of this law to address the grievances of patients were widely commented upon (Bhatt, 1996) and the need for credible, effective and satisfying alternatives have been suggested (VHAI, 1997). The national health policy 2002 recognizes the need for regulation but no tangible blueprint of regulation has emerged so far.

The issue of regulation however, is not confined to the healthcare institutions. It extends to the larger area of health laws with their inadequate and faulty provisions and tardy implementation which provide scope for evasion (Bhatt, 1996; Bose, 2002). The interventions of the apex court have forced the Government to take note of the deficiencies in this sphere. The enactment of new health laws covering organ transplants, sex determination tests and the emergence of high technology interventions involving stem cells, genetics, in-vitro fertilization, etc. which are practised without effective regulation have lent greater urgency to this matter. The experience of enforcing new health laws referred to above has already exposed their weaknesses, considering the widespread violations reported from time to time. With India becoming an attractive destination for BPOs in respect of clinical trials due to the lax regulatory regime and poverty of population as well as a preferred choice for the patients availing of sophisticated surgical interventions due to the low cost and absence of regulations covering such emergent areas becomes glaringly evident. The loopholes in existing laws and incapacity of implementing machinery to enforce them by effective inspections and meticulous efforts for prosecution of violations and securing conviction have sharply brought out the governance deficit. The discourse on the subject has also touched upon the inadequacy of investigation infrastructure—laboratories for testing samples of drugs, food samples and clinical products as well as institutional arrangements for training of personnel engaged in enforcement. The failure to address these issues has led to the extensive intervention of higher level courts in public interest litigations.

EQUITY

The equity in healthcare refers to lack of differentiation in the use of healthcare and capacity to avail of it when in need and similar availability of various determinants of health to all those who seek them so as to produce broadly equal distribution of health outcomes. Equity can be measured by a diverse range of parameters such as incidence of disease across social groups, access to and utilization of healthcare facilities, capacity to spend on health-seeking benefits, and the position regarding availability of the social determinants of health [Murlidharan, 1993; Qadeer, 1985]. Judged by these parameters, there are inequities galore which are driven by diverse factors—geographical, caste, class, religion and gender. The health status of people judged by the incidence of illness across social groups shows a huge rural-urban divide, with rural areas throwing up higher morbidity rates when compared to the urban areas. This skewness also prevails in respect of regions and communities in the country, between the rich and the poor, the upper castes and the lower castes and females as against males in both rural and urban areas. The differentiation of varying degree can also be observed in the incidence of acute ailments, chronic diseases, rates of hospitalization, untreated episodes of diseases among people located in different geographical areas and belonging to different social categories. There are sharp class differentials in utilization of health care services in public and private health sector as well as in expenditure incurred on health. The level of utilization of public healthcare services among STs was found to be more than in other sub-groups. The medical expenditure by households was the lowest among the STs, followed by SCs and others respectively. The rich spend more on healthcare than the poor. The indebtedness on account of health expenditure financing for in-patient care was 25% in the urban areas as compared to 45% in the rural areas (Dilip, 2005).

In terms of the social determinants of health such as distribution of poverty, access to safe drinking water and sanitation and status of literacy, there is not only a substantial urban and rural divide with the former showing a much better position in respect of these indices than the latter but also a huge gap across social groups. The SCs and STs fare much worse than the other social groups. A similar position obtains in respect of their access to durable employment, stable income, food security, living and working conditions and level of consumer expenditure, all of which contribute to the adverse health outcomes in respect of these groups.

Enforcing equity in health has all long been a huge challenge to governance. To meet this challenge, action was necessary not only for equitable spread of public health services but also for improving access to them by neutralizing caste, class, communal, gender, income and geographical barriers. The poor had also to be protected from falling into the debt and poverty trap due to the exorbitant out-of-pocket expenditure (in excess of 80%) on seeking treatment. The priority in attention was needed to target those who avoid seeking treatment in respect of ailments considered serious due to lack of purchasing power. This category of persons, as per a recent survey, constitute a whopping 40% of the respondents (JSA, 2009). Simultaneous action was also required for forging social determinants with a view to improving health outcomes of these vulnerable groups. This challenge was not met even in the first phase when the nature of economy was welfare-centric. These inequities have exacerbated with the onset of market-oriented transformation of health policy. The iniquities are now so widespread that a marginal increase in public health expenditure, improvement effected in public healthcare institutions with inputs of personnel, drugs, training and public private partnerships and a modicum of social insurance cover for the poorer sections would be insufficient to bridge them. To tackle this problem, structural changes in the public healthcare system to offset the impact of market forces on the functionality and quality of healthcare and a concerted attack on the key determinants of exclusion and differentiation in access would have to be taken.

MANAGEMENT

The management of the public health system is expected to ensure that all inputs are provided timely to units rendering health services in order that they function optimally and contribute to achieving the desired health outcomes. This management function involves action on two fronts—intra-sectoral and inter-sectoral. The intra-sectoral action refers to provisioning of necessary inputs for its healthcare centres to function efficiently and effectively and rendering quality service. The inter-sectoral management refers to coordination with other sectoral agencies to promote good health.

Internal Management

The internal management of the public health system assumes considerable importance since the healthcare facilities fail to function effectively because essential inputs are not available. This management function has to be exercised at all levels where health services are provided or decisions concerning them are taken—central, state, district, block and facility. But the state and district levels are crucial; the state because the key decisions are taken and funds distributed at that level and the district because it is there that the process of implementation gets initiated. The central level is, by and large, confined to the allocation of resources in respect of central grants and programmes, issuing programme guidelines and monitoring of information flowing from states about implementation of health programmes. The block level has not yet emerged as an unit of management since the district level management directly controls the facilities. The facility-level management is dependent on the support systems to function efficiently and, therefore, looks up to the district level for addressing its needs.

The function of state-level health management is carried out by the Directorate of Health Services reporting to the

Secretary, Health Department with the Minister in charge of health portfolio taking final decisions. In addition, para-statal bodies have been established to facilitate easier decision making, better coordination with the related divisions of the organization and expeditious financial transactions. The district-level health management operates under the control of a district officer, called the Chief Medical Officer (CMO) who also looks after the peripheral health facilities and national programmes. The district hospital is exclusively managed by a civil surgeon. The CMO is assisted by programme officers just as the Director, Health Services at the state level is assisted by joint/deputy directors each dealing with specific programmes. Lately, para-statal bodies have been set up at the district level also.

The management functions at both levels relate to the supervision of health facilities, provision of required inputs and support to them and implementation of specific health programmes (disease control, externally aided, etc.).

At the central level, responsibility for management of health programmes and institutions lies with the Ministry of Health and Family Welfare which is assisted by the Directorate General of Health Services (DGHS). Similar to the organizational arrangement at the state level, the DGHS reports to the Secretary, Health and Family Welfare with Minister in charge taking decisions. He functions with the help of a number of officers designated as additional, joint or deputy directors, each dealing with a programme or a subject relating to the health establishment. The Central government also administers tertiary care hospitals and institutions of medical education besides organizations devoted to medical research, investigation and vaccine production. It handles most of the externally-aided projects and matters relating to policy and planning. It is the chief agency to allocate programme funds to the state governments. The problems of governance at the central level arise from the organizational arrangement of health establishment, programme structures, health planning process and approach to the diversity of medicine systems. Some of these issues are briefly discussed below.

Organization of the health policy establishment

The organization of health establishment at the Central and state levels is crucial to the efficient and effective functioning of health programmes and healthcare institutions and attending to other matters relating to health. The problems arise when this structural arrangement gets fragmented leading to difficulties in addressing the policy and programme issues in a coordinated and focused manner. This fragmentation emerged at the Central level when a separate department from the erstwhile unified Ministry of Health was carved out to deal with family planning and associated MCH and RCH programmes. This bifurcation delinked primary healthcare from the rest of health problems and created enormous coordination difficulties. It also distorted the perspective of primary healthcare as well as of women's health. The process of fragmentation proceeded further when yet another department dealing with the Indian Systems of Medicine and Homoeopathy (ISM&H) was created. Though the arrangement was made to devote greater attention to these systems of medicine, this has not helped in judicious availability of the ISM&H treatment at the primary healthcare level. More recently, the subject of medical research has been split to constitute an additional department of the Ministry. The latest development in the organizational arrangement is the formation of a separate department exclusively dealing with HIV-AIDS. This carries further the anachronistic arrangement of having a separate National AIDS Control Organization at the behest of the World Bank. All these organizational arrangements adversely affect the availability of services at the primary healthcare since forging of horizontal convergence of inputs from these departments with separate hierarchies of command and control would be an uphill task for any management.

At the level of the State, fragmentation has taken the form of separate para-statal bodies, called the State health societies each dealing with separate disease control programme funded by the external agencies. These para-statal agencies fragment the process of decision making, divest the political head of the organization of control and, therefore, dilute his capacity to issue directions for efficient management of programmes and institutions. This arrangement also makes decision making less accountable.

Another important issue of the health organization relates to the total absence of public health experience in those who preside over the health policy planning and execution in the Central government. The top medical professionals in the Directorate General of Health Services are all drawn from teaching and research institutions and central hospitals and are specialists in their disciplines. They are, therefore, not rooted in the healthcare problems of people in villages and small towns as well as in the preventive work (Jeffrey, 1988). Their perspective is shaped by developments in the field of medicine at the international level. They are frequently involved in international consultations pertaining to their specialty and many of them go over to the international institutions after retirement as consultants, advisors, etc. Their views and approaches to health problems are easily moulded by ideas and proposals coming from foreign agencies and have no grounding in how they would work in the context of our rural situation. The total revamping of the recruitment policy for such positions so as to have public health experts in them has often been raised.

Other issues of organizational nature in the Central and state governments relate to the concentration of authority, multiple structures, overlapping work, lack of coordination and accountability and inefficient utilization of available human and institutional resources (Mishra et al., 2003). Recently, the Government of India has merged the Family Welfare Department with the Health Department. The separate health societies at State and district levels have been amalgamated into a single society. But there is little else by way of efficient reorganization that has come about at the state or central levels.

Health planning

As per the Constitution, the exclusive jurisdiction of the Central government relates only to the national institutions in medical education and research. Public health and sanitation, hospitals and dispensaries are in the State list. Medical education, drugs, family planning, control of inter-state communicable diseases, mental health and medical professions are in the Concurrent list. But the Central government has increasingly encroached upon the state jurisdiction and exercised a larger role in health planning since Independence. This centralization is the result of internal as well as external factors. The internal factors include the system of transfer of financial resources from Central government to state governments for development activities, besides what the states are able to generate through their own efforts. The funds for development activities are provided by the Central government through the Planning Commission, centrally-sponsored schemes with 100% or less assistance, public health programmes relating to immunization, disease control and family planning. Centralization is also exercised through expertise built up in national institutions of investigation and research which lay down parameters for implementation of all health programmes and their diagnostic and treatment regimen. The central control is equally manifested in determining prioritization of health programmes, their design, strategy and delivery system (Mishra et al., 2003). The Central government has derived these powers by drawing upon the Concurrent list as also with the implicit consent of the state governments. The centralization in health governance has been specifically promoted and expanded by the externally-aided projects. Starting with the Malaria control programme right from its inception, the list of such projects included other major disease control programes of TB, Leprosy and public health programmes relating to immunization and maternal and child health. Later, HIV-AIDS and blindness control got added to this list. The externally-aided projects created centralized and verticalized structures of programme management with little autonomy to the states for making any changes.

This centralization of health planning has come in for a great deal of criticism because of the distortions it has created in respect of the prioritization of health programmes, resource allocation, design of decision-making structures, etc. The externally financed disease control programmes have also been severely critiqued for being techno-centric. The methodology of their selection is not based on the available epidemiological information and social dimensions of diseases, their distribution and linkages (Banerjee, 1999) but on the effectiveness of technological intervention and efficiency of financial investment (Priya, 2001[a]). These programmes have also been questioned for shifting the focus from diseases of the poor of the Third World to the priority in the disease profile of the industrialized world and their choice of technology and institutional control [Qadeer, 1995; ICSSR-ICMR; 1981; VHAI, 1997].

The centralization in health planning has yet another adverse impact. It fails to generate ownership of programmes among the state governments, which impacts on their implementation. It also tends to divert financial and manpower resources from states' own health priorities to the ones set by the Central government. This loss of state autonomy has led to a progressive weakening of the capacity and confidence of the healthcare providers and decision makers at the state level in tackling health emergencies and their increasing dependence upon Central directives and technical assistance.

The centralization of health planning has been held responsible for creating bottlenecks in the implementation of programmes. This arises from their restructured financial management reflected in the pattern of flow of resources from the Centre to the states with its multiple checks and uncertainties, absence of advance intimation regarding allocation, rigid budgetary controls and insistence on the provision of state share for release of central funds, etc. [Satia et al., 1999; Bhatt, 1999]. These centralizing tendencies have created severe tensions within the health organization. The problems of governance resulting from them largely remain confined to the discourse within the health organization and rarely spill over to the public domain to permit greater exposure to the adverse impact they create on the public health system.

Structures of health programmes

The sharpest critique in the discourse on health relates to the distorted organizational arrangements and priorities in health programmes. This is manifested in the excessive emphasis on Family Planning (now Welfare) Programme at the behest of international agencies (Banerjee, 1999) which completely eclipses other programmes in primary healthcare (Jeffrey, 1988). The concentration of resources and manpower on this programme has led to the relative neglect of other healthcare needs and priorities emerging from the available information on disease profile and other health problems. The discourse on family planning (welfare) programme itself has extensively dwelt on the strategy of implementation with coercive overtones, monitoring methods fixated on target orientation, failure to follow up cases, deficiency in addressing unmet needs and omission to attend to the numerous health problems of women unconnected with reproductive health, all of which have a bearing on the governance dimensions. The other distortion has been introduced by way of separate and vertical disease control programmes which violate the composite nature of primary healthcare, adversely affect the access of people to programme benefits and lead to inefficient use of financial and manpower resources.

The neglect of public health in overall health planning caused by the prioritization of disease control and family planning programmes has also featured in the studies on the health system. The preventive aspects of diseases have been progressively neglected, except for the immunization programme. Health planning has failed to sufficiently focus on sanitation, drinking water, infection control, environmental management, etc. in terms of allocation of resources, provision of sufficient manpower, capacity building and inter-sectoral convergence (Dasgupta, 2005). The campaign mode of implementation of certain programmes (for example, Pulse Polio) has also been widely criticized for creating distortions in the use of resources—human, financial and institutional, leading to the neglect of other health problems of the people. The failure to respond to these issues by restructured health organization and programmes and revamped health planning with corresponding interventions is indicative of the state of governance in this sector.

Medicinal Systems

Sub-optimal utilization

The public health facilities in the ISM&H streams are fairly large. These systems have 23,597 dispensaries and 6,88,802 registered practitioners (Planning Commission, 2002). Nearly 21,974 ISM&H doctors are working in the PHCs. This huge infrastructure is under-utilized. This is on account of the failure of management at the Central and state levels. The system also faces bias from health planning establishment which is dominated by professionals from the allopathic stream of medicine. The inability to integrate the ISM&H steams with the Western (allopathic) health system is attributed to lack of objective evaluation of its contribution. The ISM&H segment of healthcare system suffers from numerous problems. These include cross-practice by its doctors, irrational distribution of facilities, domination of commercial preparations in prescription, absence of standard treatment protocols, quality-related parameters of drug production and a list of essential drugs at the state level, inadequate budget allocation, insufficient emphasis on training, skill upgradation, monitoring and supervision and failure to improve the quality of medical education. Overall, the public health system displays lack of requisite political will and imagination to make optimal and effective use of the available infrastructure and resources of these streams.

Skewed development

The dominance of the Western system of medicine and neglect of Indian systems of medicine and homoeopathy leading to imbalanced development and use of the two segments has been raised by the civil society organizations, votaries of the alternative medicine and critics of the public health system. The discourse has focused on the bias in allocation of resources, low level of utilization of large manpower and institutional facilities, inadequate opportunities for their development, lack of efforts for improving standards of their education, training and drug production and reluctance to mainstream these systems in the primary healthcare. The major sore point has been the inability of the Government to synthesize various systems of medicine in the curricula of medical education and treatment of illness for the benefit of people (Mishra et al., 2003). With the coming into existence of a separate department dealing with the ISM&H, the issues concerning improvement in standards of education and drug production are receiving attention particularly in the wake of interest shown by the Western countries in these systems (MoHFW 2002[b]; Planning Commission, 2002). But the larger issue of the ISM&H streams continuing to remain a peripheral unit of the overall public health system and health organization of the country remains unaddressed.

The critics have also highlighted lack of will and efforts to nurture Indian traditions in folk medicine despite people's acceptance of them, and failure to mainstream them on the basis of community evaluation. The recurring campaign of Western medicine to castigate folk medicine as quackery is leading to the growing loss of confidence among the practitioners, reluctance to pass on talent to the members of the family and gradual disappearance of this valuable treasure of knowledge (Shankar, 2001). The Government has failed to take any action to preserve, encourage and appropriately use this folk medical knowledge.

Inputs

Since the institutions of primary healthcare fall in the domain of state governments, the problems relating to their management are experienced at the state level. Some of these problems relate to inputs such as human resource management, procurement and maintenance, orientation of medical education, diverse medicine system and health system research. These are briefly discussed here.

Human Resource Management

Availability of Personnel

The greatest challenge to governance in the health sector has been to ensure that service providers are available in the healthcare facilities. The non-functionality of primary healthcare has been attributed largely to the absence from duty of doctors, specialists and paramedics. This situation is primarily due to the unwillingness of these personnel, particularly the doctors and the specialists, to work in the rural areas. The urban background, hospital-based nature of their training and high level of professional and lifestyle aspirations contribute to this bias against rural postings (Gautham, 2006). The Government has sought to tackle this problem through a number of incentives and disincentives. But this approach has not worked to change the attitude of health personnel (Jeffrey, 1988). The problem continues to linger despite the huge number of doctors produced in the public and private sector medical colleges (Planning Commission, 2002). The discourse on health has highlighted this problem all along. But there has been no effective solution in sight. In the post-reforms period, efforts were made to engage healthcare providers from the private sector facilities on contract to get over this difficulty. But the arrangement has not worked because the under-served rural areas, where the problem is most acute, also do not have private sector medical facilities or qualified practitioners. The feasibility of this arrangement is in doubt on other grounds as well. The NRHM has taken note of this deficiency to address the problem. It is proposed to make a two-year stint in the rural healthcare units compulsory for all medical graduates before they get their qualifying degree. This has been stoutly opposed by the students pursuing medical education and there have been agitations in some parts of the country against this decision. In the short run, the Government is relying on getting services from the private sector, utilizing general duty practitioners for specialist work after short duration training for some specialties and AYUSH doctors against non-specialist vacancies. But these ad hoc solutions do not address the basic issue of unsuitability of medical education.

Private practice

The private practice resorted to by doctors employed in the public health system, a trend started during the colonial period, has adversely affected the efficiency and quality of the services delivered (Baru, 1995). It also tells upon the integrity of the personnel involved. This has given rise to several unethical practices. The doctors absent themselves from their rural postings to carry on their private practice in the urban areas. They neglect their duties in the public health facilities, and use resources of the public hospitals to benefit patients accessing their private facilities (Jessani and Anantharaman, 1993). They are also known to direct patients accessing the public health facilities to seek services in their private clinics/hospitals and provide services in public hospitals for patients registered in their private clinics. This obnoxious practice has been extensively critiqued in the discourse on health. State governments across the country have attempted to abolish private practice but have met with little success due to stiff resistance from the doctors and the political clout they command (Baru, 1998). The expansion of private sector facilities has made no dent in this arrangement. The Central government, has, however, succeeded in enforcing a ban on the private practice by doctors employed in its health facilities by providing the incentive of additional pay. But the Central government hospitals are located in the urban areas. This incentive is unlikely to work in the rural areas and small towns where surveillance is difficult. It has not worked in respect of the state government doctors even in the state capital. The state governments are virtually reconciled to the current situation. The issue continues to pose the toughest challenge to governance.

Training

The absence of durable arrangements for periodic training of the doctors to update their knowledge has been persistently raised by the experts and also recognized by the medical professionals themselves. Even in respect of the doctors employed in the public health system at the primary healthcare level, there is no arrangement for such periodic training. Only short-term and ad hoc training is arranged in respect of those deployed for implementation of the externally aided, specific disease control and immunization programmes (Mavalankar, 1999). This training, however, is limited to imparting knowledge about clinical and administrative guidelines crucial to their implementation. There are neither programmes nor institutional arrangements where periodic training can be imparted for enabling doctors and specialists in the rural healthcare institutions to update their knowledge about the fast pace of advances in the field of medicine. The medical councils are expected to ensure that the private practitioners update their knowledge and to arrange programmes for imparting it. But this does not happen. The associations of medical professionals have also failed to arrange training for their members. In this situation, the onus is on the medical professionals themselves to update their knowledge through their individual efforts. This becomes difficult due to lack of access to experts, hospitals and relevant literature. As a result, there is a progressive loss of self-confidence among the medical practitioners employed in the public health system which leads to the tendency of unwarranted transfer of patients to referral institutions and specialists and incidence of faulty diagnosis and treatment. The situation in respect of training is even more acute in respect of the practitioners of ISM&H whether in the Government or the private sector. The problem is recognized by the Government. The NRHM has made a provision for training and skill development for registered medical practitioners to help them improve their skills in the framework for implementation and the states are encouraged to arrange it (Sinha, 2009). It has to seen whether any credible arrangement for such training has emerged.

Behaviour of service providers

The behavioural problems of healthcare providers are also responsible for low utilization of public health services, particularly in the rural areas. The typical experience of a patient accessing a health facility, even in the urban areas (considerably more in the rural areas) is the disinclination of the attending doctor to listen to the patient [Palaniswamy, 2006], impatience to dispose of him/her, refusal to take into account personal and social aspects of illness, shouting at the patient if he/she persists with his/her queries, unhelpful attitude to sort out difficulties faced in accessing services, etc. (Patnaik, 2005; Das et al., 2004). The complaints against lower level health personnel include even cheating, manipulation and extracting illegal gratification for extending entitled benefits. The SC/ST patients also experience caste bias in the behaviour of providers in the rural areas. In the case of women, lack of privacy in attending to their complaints, and dismissal of their perception and experience of disease and its social construction in the context of gender relations are frequently encountered. These dimensions of behaviour are all related to the attitude, value system and social bias of service providers and have been highlighted by the health activists and researchers. Yet, in the delivery of public healthcare, behaviour of providers is the least recognized and the most neglected governance problem. There is little by way of response from the Government in terms of training and orientation of health personnel and restructuring of programmes and operational facilities to address these concerns.

Cadre Management

The problems associated with management of cadres of healthcare providers, particularly doctors and specialists, have also surfaced in the health discourse from time to time (Mishra et al., 2003). These include lack of transparency and adherence to norms in postings and transfers of medical personnel, (Reddy et al., 2006), mismatch in deployment of medical personnel reflected in such distortions as placement of doctors in excess of the sanctioned strength in more developed areas as against short of such strength in underserved ones, placement of specialists against general duty posts, failure to effect timely promotions, laxity in taking disciplinary action against doctors who absent themselves from notified postings (Gill and Ghuman, 2000), as also those who overstay abroad despite directives to return and to effectively pursue complaints of negligence, unethical practices, misgovernance, corruption, etc. Most of these issues are usually discussed within the Government and do not get much exposure in the public domain. A major reason for this inefficient management can be attributed to the centralization of cadres of health personnel which creates enormous difficulties in exercising control over them and making them accountable to the people.

The centralized recruitment, deployment, promotion and disciplinary control of various categories of healthcare providers have created conditions for extensive political influence in the management of their cadres (Satia et al., 1999). The problems associated with centralized cadre management include lack of transparency and norm-based deployment of health personnel (Mishra et al., 2003), delay in recruitment and promotion against available vacancies, use of political elite by influential medical personnel to get desired postings or seek reversal of unfavourable decisions in this regard (Jeffrey, 1988) and worst of all, erosion of accountability of the healthcare providers to the local officials and community where they are posted. These issues have all along figured in the literature on health sector governance but have come up more sharply after the restructuring of panchayati raj institutions. The centralized cadre management of health officials is among the more important explanations for the inability of panchayati raj bodies to effectively use powers and resources devolved on them for the benefit of their constituents and to enforce accountability of the service providers in their jurisdiction. While this issue continues to be highlighted by the civil society organizations, the management of cadres of health personnel continues to elude any systemic reform.

Procurement and Maintenance

Procurement of drugs

The non-availability of drugs in the public health units has been a recurring complaint of the patients accessing them, which is responsible for low utilization of services provided therein. This has been recognized in the National Health Policy, 2002 and elsewhere in policy documents (MoHFW, 2002[a]; Planning Commission, 2002). The insufficient allocation has been cited as a major reason for this deficiency. The critique of the public health system has invariably referred to this problem and a higher budgetary allocation to meet the deficiency has been advocated. But what has usually been missed in the analysis of this issue is that even the funds available for procurement of drugs, though admittedly inadequate, are not judiciously utilized. This is due to the faulty procurement system. Therefore, the governance problems relating to procurement of drugs contribute substantially to their non-availability to the patients. The reform of procurement system did not receive sufficient attention in the pre-reforms period. Lately, the World Bank has raised this issue in a big way and even financed projects for a restructured procurement system in some states (Mishra et al., 2003).

Governance issues arise when drugs already purchased and supplied to the health facilities are not used because: (a) there is a mismatch between the demand and supply—drugs needed are not supplied, while those supplied are not needed and, therefore, remain unused and get wasted. There is also no efficient arrangement to transfer such drugs to facilities where they may be needed; (b) drugs are received in the health units after considerable delay and almost nearing their expiry date resulting in their non-utilization thereafter. Both these problems point to a defective procurement and distribution system. The other problems relate to purchase of substandard drugs from lesser known suppliers apparently influenced by the lowest price offer, political interference/bureaucratic corruption, centralized procurement, storage and distribution resulting in bottlenecks, incapacity to negotiate with standard suppliers for procurement of drugs at reasonable rates, absence of an approved list of standard essential drugs, etc. The governance problems in respect of procurement of drugs are on account of the failure to put in place a standardized and transparent system of procurement with a comprehensive manual prescribing step-by-step process of action. In some states, a greater problem lies in the reluctance of officials charged with this responsibility to take decisions relating to procurement lest allegations of corruption, favouritism and unfair dealings in transactions are raised and an enquiry is ordered which may cause harassment to them. This problem is directly related to lack of a fool proof system which brooks no interference and leaves no room for any bias. The deficit of confidence in taking procurement decisions is also due to lack of knowledge about drugs and its composition, cost of manufacture, the prominent manufacturers/suppliers, the rationale for cost differential of the same drug manufactured by different agencies, market profile and negotiation skills to extract a reasonable price offer. These issues have now figured in a big way in the discourse on health governance at the official level. The Tamil Nadu project for procurement and distribution of drugs, where a specialized agency has been exclusively set up for this work, has been cited as a way to deal with these issues.

Governance issues also relate to enforcing laws to check spurious and hazardous drugs, training of doctors in the practice of rational medicine, breaking the nexus between drug companies and doctors in prescription practice, controlling the pattern of drug production to disallow numerous irrational and expensive combinations, preparing and circulating a list of essential drugs, regulating prices of drugs to check huge profit margins, etc. (Locost, 2004; VHAI, 1997). These issues have been vigorously raised by the consumer organizations and public interest advocacy groups with little coming by way of tangible response from the Government so far. In the pre-reforms period, some interventions were made to control prices of essential drugs and set up public sector production units to make essential drugs available at reasonable prices. The de-regulation drive in the post-reforms period has reversed these decisions. The vacuum thus created has provided space for citizens to approach the higher courts to intervene and issue directions to the Government to protect them from irrational prices of drugs fixed by the manufacturing companies.

Functioning equipments

The non-functioning equipments in public health facilities contribute to their low utilization, besides causing irritation and inconvenience to the patients. This happens because of several factors. Quite often, there is a failure to evolve a proper system for purchase, repair and maintenance of equipments. The problems relating to purchase of equipments include failure to evaluate the cost and benefits of different choices and go in for the most cost-effective equipment. With regard to the selection of equipments, the usual bias is in favour of foreign brands and opting for expensive and latest technology without giving weightage to cost, frequency of use and difficulties associated with operation, maintenance and repair. In respect of maintenance and repairs, the problems can be attributed to the failure to conclude contracts timely and insert necessary clauses in them relating to prompt and cost-effective service. There is also negligence in invoking the warranty clause in time. The equipments going out of order are not peculiar to the public health system though it may happen there more often due to frequency of use. But the failure to get them repaired or replaced within a reasonable time is observed more often in the public health facilities. The centralized decision making for ordering repairs is an important reason for the enormous delay in setting them right. Inadequate funds often constrain efforts in seeking timely repair for even minor breakdowns by the health units themselves. The absence of a local agent of supplier, particularly in the case of foreign equipments, increases both cost and delay in attending to the complaints. The lack of circumspection on these and other related aspects prior to the purchase of equipments has been responsible for making inefficient choices. (Griffiths, 1980; Murlidharan, 2001).

Governance problems also extend to equipments already procured but lying idle for a long time. This is because necessary preparatory work (construction of a room, air-conditioning of the premises) to install them have not been done in time or the operators have not been trained or recruited. The non-functioning equipments could, at times, be a manipulated phenomenon due to the nexus of doctors/decision makers with private diagnostic agencies in order that the patients could be referred to the latter who, in turn, provide a commission for this purpose. There is also a tendency for the public health establishments to prefer replacement of equipment over its repair. This causes delay because the purchase of equipment requires sufficient funds to be allocated and procedural formalities to be observed before the order for purchase is given. These issues figure prominently as administrative problems in the discourse within the public health system though they may not be so widely known outside the Government.

Orientation of Medical Education

The elite orientation of medical education has been extensively commented upon by perceptive health experts, researchers and social activists (Madan, 1980; Banerjee, 1996). The unsuitability of medical education to national requirements has been attributed to its urban orientation, techno-centric bias, emphasis on specialization, focus on diseases of the industrial world and indifference to public and community health. The disinclination of the doctors to work in the rural areas has also been related to these reasons (Oomen, 1987). The curricula, mode of training and the system of selection for entrants to the course are responsible for this state of medical education. The curricula is exclusively hospital based and patient oriented and ignores entirely the social causation of disease. The training focuses on analytical approach from symptoms to physical examination to laboratory diagnosis and treatment which is unsuited to the rural areas where limited diagnostic aids and range of therapy has to adopted taking into account the deficiencies of infrastructure as well as social conditions of the patient (Sen, 1975). The selection process is weighted in favour of public school education, puts premium on academic success to the neglect of attitudes, values and motives. The critics, in desperation, have, therefore, suggested a shift in the pattern of health manpower production with exclusive focus on the rural areas to overcome this problem.

In the past, attempts have been made to introduce community and public health focus in medical education with rural attachment. This is like treating gangrene with lavender water. Obviously, it has had little impact on the outlook of medical students since there is neither any radical change in the curricula nor in the approach to training and the process of selection of entrants. The need for extensive reorientation of medical education has featured in the discourse on health governance (Bajaj, 1998). The Tenth Five-Year Plan and the National Rural Health Mission have also reflected this sentiment (Planning Commission, 2002; MoHFW, 2005). Nothing by way of restructured medical education has emerged in this regard so far.

Health Systems Research

The importance of research in public health as input to the management of health system is not recognized. This explains the virtual absence of such a research at the state and district levels which could provide analysis of the medical and social determinants of diseases encountered in primary healthcare. Those responsible for health planning and programme implementation at the state level consider such a research unnecessary and a purely academic activity to be undertaken by specialized institutions. Their attention is entirely focused on action (PHRN, 2006). Due to this negative attitude, no comprehensive analysis of diseases afflicting people in different areas, their epidemiological and qualitative dimensions, group and location, specific characteristics is available to the health practitioners and the planners. They are, consequently, deprived of these insights for designing of suitable measures, preventive and curative, for dealing with them which is effective, cost efficient and locally relevant. Also, in the absence of a provision of research, much-needed information does not get collected and a valuable experience gathered during practice in the districts gets wasted. As doctors are transferred from one area to another, the new incumbents to the job get no help from past efforts in dealing with the same set of health problems. The health establishment is satisfied with providing curative treatment when illness occurs. The investment in research infrastructure is considered unnecessary and even wasteful. State officials depend upon central research institutions for assistance when they are unable to control the eruption of a disease with uncommon characteristics or unresponsive to standard treatment. But the nature of research is different at different levels. Central specialized research institutions should confine themselves to complex research problems with cross-country dimensions and global ramifications. Public health research is best handled at the district and state level due to easy access to information, better understanding of the area and people and cost efficiency of its operations. But there seems to be no indication that this truth has been realized.

Management—Inter-sectoral

Social Determinants of Health

The health policy crafted after Independence had an integrated view of health incorporating its social determinants—sanitation, drinking water, poverty alleviation (employment), nutrition, social security, etc. (Bose and Desai, 1983). This integration, however, failed to get incorporated in the structure of health services. The social development programmes focusing on these supportive elements were and continue to be implemented by separate agencies with no linkages to the health problems. The lack of needed convergence pursuant to the objectives and approaches enshrined in the health policy has been a recurring criticism in the discourse on the health system (Mishra et al., 2003). The agencies dealing with health are structurally weak and deficient in conceptual approach and institutional arrangements for effecting this convergence. The allocation of subjects in the rules of business in the Central and state governments is also responsible for this inadequacy because the activities of the Ministry/Department relating to health are limited to healthcare aspects and not extended to the broader view of health. The lack of seriousness in pursuing this theme in the overall health planning and delivery of health programmes continues to exist. This is despite increasing evidence of the adverse health outcomes arising from the inability of health agencies to forge links with social developments programmes. The National Rural Health Mission has committed to take some action in this direction by devolving on the village health and sanitation committee the responsibility of integrating health care with sanitation, etc. But this tokenistic arrangement is totally inadequate to the complexity of task. The integration, to be effective, has to start from the apex level, i.e., the Government of India where development activities which promote good health are dealt with by different ministries which have their sectoral schemes and programmes. There is no agency forging their integration to achieve optimal health outcomes. This fragmentation percolates down to state and district levels. Therefore, this structural bottleneck has to be neutralized. The approach to such integration has to be designed and institutional arrangements created for effecting it at various levels. There is no indication that this is happening.

Social Control

Community Participation

The importance of community participation was emphasized in the very first articulation of health policy after Independence for ensuring better reach of services and enforcing accountability of service providers. There was, however, a lack of interest and efforts in giving effect to it. The bureaucratic/technocratic structures were the preferred mode of implementation of health programmes. This came in for strong criticism from experts, social scientists as well as the civil society organizations. The critics attributed the neglect of community participation to the indifference of service providers and absence of political commitment. This is typically reflected in the approach to community participation which treated community as a helping agent in carrying out programme directives from above rather than an active partner in designing and executing programmes (ICSSR–ICMR, 1981; Rifkin, 1985).

The earliest attempt for facilitating community participation was made through the community development programme of the 1950s which covered within its ambit the entire gamut of rural development—agriculture, cooperatives, education, health, etc. Its failure to achieve the objective has been extensively researched and documented. In any case, this programme did not focus on health specifically. The initiative for effecting community participation specific to health services was made in the late 1970s with the introduction of 'community health worker' at the village level in the primary healthcare. The collapse of this experiment within a few years of its introduction has been attributed to lack of political commitment to the objective and the hostility of medical professionals to transfer knowledge to these workers and repose trust in the arrangement. The techno-centric disease control programmes have not even made a pretence of incorporating community participation in their design and schematic arrangements. These programmes have also bypassed the panchayati raj institutions in their structures of implementation. The governance in public health system has remained lukewarm to the involvement of community and democratic bodies at the grassoots level while paying lip service to participation. However, the recently launched NRHM incorporates an assurance to involve the panchayati raj bodies in the health programmes at the primary healthcare level. It has also made Accredited Social Health Activist (ASHA) at the village level the sheet anchor of community participation. But the larger governance issues relating to community participation raised in the civil society critique (ICSSR-ICMR, 1981) still remain unaddressed. Even the ASHA experiment has raised a number of questions about the representative character of the person chosen to discharge this role and the processes through which participation of community is sought to be realized.

Decentralization

As indicated earlier, centralization has been the bane of health planning. The verticalization of Disease Control Programmes has strengthened this tendency. The centralized and hierarchical health organization contributes to this practice. The expansion of Central government's role in the health system facilitates this process. To counteract these centralizing trends, decentralization of both health planning and health organization has been recommended. This decentralization would promote effective, efficient and transparent delivery of services which would contribute to more responsive healthcare and greater social accountability. It has been one of the key governance reforms the importance of which has been recognized even in the Common Review Mission Report of the NRHM (NRHM–2007). In the earlier phase, decentralization was conceived in terms of larger financial allocation, greater delegation of power and authority of decision making and transfer of administrative control over healthcare units and health officials from the level of the state to the level of district and below. The association of village community with health programmes and involvement of Panchayati Raj Institutions in their implementation were also suggested. But there was little by way of concrete institutionalization of these ideas. With the 73rd amendment to the Constitution, the PRIs have emerged as a third tier of the Government which have a defined domain of the specified areas of development. Health is one of the subjects in the list of sectoral activities earmarked for them. Still, nothing of consequence happened to empower the PRIs in the health sector in line with the 73rd amendment. Recently, the NRHM has recognized the need for mainstreaming the strategic role of the PRIs in the management of public health services and implementation of public health programmes. However, it has conceived this strategic role of the PRIs in terms of providing a representation to the PRIs in management bodies or consulting them in processes of decision making. The measures through which the PRIs have been involved in the structures and processes of implementation of the NRHM consist of village health and sanitation committees, opening of joint accounts for management of untied fund at the sub-Centre level, block and district-level health missions. The Rogi Kalyan Samities at the PHC, CHC, sub-district and district-level health facilities also have representation of the PRIs. The PRIs are also to be consulted before the approval of the district health plan. The other steps envisaged are delegation of power of recruitment of contractual staff to the block or district panchayats, transfer of ownership of Sub Centres and PHCs to the panchayats and devolution of adequate resources and administrative support to them for this purpose. The preparation of a district health plan and village health plan are also modes of implementing the commitment towards decentralization. On substantive issues like transfer of ownership of health facilities and control over service providers, little progress has been achieved. The district-level health planning is still at a processual stage to permit its impact on the centralized health plan. The fundamental issue of transfer of requisite powers of decision making, allocation of sufficient financial resources and administrative control over health staff and facilities consistent with the responsibilities envisaged in the 73rd amendment continues to face strong resistance from political as well as bureaucratic interests. The decentralized planning and implementation of primary healthcare cannot even begin without dismantling the centralized structures of planning and state management of health facilities and cadres of health service providers. Effecting genuine decentralization, therefore, remains a challenging task.

Accountability

The issue of accountability of health service providers is closely linked to the issue of decentralization of healthcare arrangements because genuine accountability can only emerge in decentralized governance.

The discourse on health largely focused on public-funded health system in the pre-reforms period. The accountability in this sector was conceived in terms of efficient functioning of the health facilities as per standards of treatment and their responsiveness to the needs of the service-seeking population. Two facets of accountability are involved here—clinical and political. The clinical accountability is viewed in terms of the rationality of treatment, adherence to its sequential regimen and adequate care of patients. This facet of accountability did not emerge as a significant issue during this period. The mystification of medical knowledge and great trust reposed in treating doctors prevented patients who were victims of negligence in the public health facilities from raising the issue. This explains why the public-funded health system has not come up with standard treatment protocols as a benchmark against which accountability of healthcare providers could be fixed. The political accountability was judged by its responsiveness to address the health problems of people. This aspect of accountability did emerge as a major issue in the primary health care. The political accountability of the health service providers was achieved when concerns were raised about the deficiencies in the existing public health units such as the absentee doctors, shortage of staff, insensitive behaviour, non-availability of drugs, non-existence of healthcare facilities in un-served areas or the failure to control virulent illness episodes involving large population or the inability to cope with chronic health problems in an area, etc. The critics advocated democratic control over the health personnel, facilities and programmes as a means of exercising this accountability. The Panchayati Raj Institutions and members of State legislature should be associated with any mechanism designed for this purpose. This aspect acquired greater thrust with the 73rd amendment to the Constitution.

The transfer of powers, resources and control over cadres of health workers to the PRIs for facilitating accountability has emerged as a major issue now. The initiative for devolution of powers, resources and authority to the PRIs taken by the Kerala government is a significant step in effecting political accountability of rural public health services. However, the exclusion of externally-funded projects from the ambit of political accountability continues to figure as a sore point because these projects cover major curative programmes in rural primary healthcare. Besides, the PRIs have no say in designing health programmes as per their need or to make modifications in the programmes conceived and planned at the Central and state levels. In fact, even the state legislature and central parliament has little effective say in respect of health programmes emerging from global health institutions and initiatives. The NRHM has initiated the exercise of preparing district health plans. The PRIs are to be consulted before their approval. To what extent these plans would reflect the needs of the people and whether these plans influence state and central health plans can also be assessed once the exercise has been accomplished. Thus, political accountability for all practical purposes is non-existent at present though certain deficiencies in the healthcare facilities and negligence of the service providers working therein are raised by the members in State and Central legislature.

The absence of clinical accountability in the public health system, however, has, of late, become very acute in the urban areas in view of the frequent cases of negligence alleged by the relatives of victims and the resultant public outburst of anger against the doctors involved as reported in the media. The situation in the rural areas could even be worse though lack of awareness may prevent such violent expressions of discontent. The absence of patient welfare organizations and reach of the media are an important factor in failure to raise the issue of clinical accountability in the rural areas. While a small beginning has been made under the NRHM for laying down the Indian public health standards of infrastructure for a 24-hour PHC and services to be provided therein, no standard protocols of treatment have yet been prepared. Even in terms of the infrastructure and services to be provided, the public health standards for a 24-hour CHC are not yet in place. The greater challenge, however, would be to effectuate these standards in the operation of services. There is, therefore, a very long way to traverse in the area of clinical accountability. The issue of accountability, both clinical and political, in the private sector healthcare is linked to the issue of regulation which has emerged as a huge area of concern.

Health Education

The importance of health education in preventive and curative care, efficient utilization of services and enforcing accountability of the healthcare providers is undisputed. Still, it is a highly neglected area in the healthcare system. The public health organization does have dedicated apex-level health education bodies both at the Central and state levels for this work. But the potential of these bodies remains underutilized and impact negligible. The discourse on health governance has attributed the low priority given to health education to the less attractive nature of the job for healthcare providers and lack of sufficient demand from the people. The critique of health governance has also exposed lack of seriousness in imparting health education to the citizens. This is evident from the unwillingness of the state governments to fill up posts of the Multi Purpose Health Workers who are primarily responsible for carrying out this work. Whatever little health education is carried out suffers from serious flaws. It is programme-centric in content and fragmented in approach. The mode of health education typically represents the hierarchical nature of communication between the providers and the people (ICSSR-ICMR, 1981). There is absence of requisite professional commitment to this work and failure to involve the PRIs and community organizations in it besides lack of efforts to provide back-up effective referral support. No serious, systemic and sustained initiatives have been forthcoming to meet these deficiencies. The NRHM expects ASHA to impart health education to the village community. It is also engaged in efforts to improve referral support.

Chapter 3

Health Sector Reforms: Impact on Governance

The reforms introduced in the macro-economic management of the country unleashed new developments which had a significant bearing on the governance in the health sector. The foremost among these factors was the new policy environment which shifted the paradigm of economy from its 'welfare' orientation to a market-driven thrust. This led to the curtailment in social expenditure and opening up of the economy to competition from private sector players, national and international. The existing pattern of state-provided social services began to be diluted, curtailed and, in some cases, dismantled. The increasing commitment to integrate with the global economy facilitated deeper penetration of MNCs in finance, investment and trade. The health sector could not remain untouched by these changes and was, in fact, a significant arena of influencing policy process and institutional arrangements in line with them. The state was in no position to resist these pressures given the economic circumstances in which liberalization was introduced. The result was declining autonomy in designing a health policy suited to the interests of people (the larger sections comprising the poor) and lesser assertiveness to implement equity-oriented measures. The governance in the public health system had to come to terms with this new policy environment. The significant new development directly relevant to the health sector was the emergence of the private health sector as the dominant supplier of services leaving public sector healthcare way behind. The private health sector now poses a formidable challenge to health governance because of the clout it has acquired in the economy. It is particularly strong in the healthcare segment and pharmaceuticals. Healthcare is, therefore, increasingly getting commodified and has, in fact, turned out to be one of the fastest growing sectors of the national economy. This development is changing its essential 'service' orientation. The liberalization imperative has also forced the Government to notify a new pharmaceutical policy which is geared to the growth of the drug industry rather than to achieving the goals of health policy. The participation of India in the new international trade regime with the World Trade Organization (WTO) as its governance structure is a corollary of its integration with the global economic order. One of its multilateral trade agreements, GATS-1995 has, for the first time, included 'services' in the ambit of trade. Health is included as one of such services. India has, therefore, opened up the health sector for international trade to harness the competitive advantage it offers in certain segments under different modes (WTO, 1995). This implies that India would have to abide by the directions of the WTO and to change laws, regulations and policies which impede free trade. The WTO is also a highly empowered body, unlike its predecessor. Its power to impose sanctions on defaulting members ensures compliance of its decisions. The trade in health services has promoted corporatization of healthcare. This has impacted on the cost and quality of and access to healthcare in general and produced unfavourable externalities for public health sector in particular. The other multilateral trade agreement most relevant to the health sector concerns the intellectual property rights called the TRIPS, the adherence to which has already led to a radical revision of the patent law and increased control of the multinational pharmaceutical companies on the drug sub-sector. This has a deleterious effect on the availability of drugs and national production, distribution and pricing of drugs coming within the ambit of patents. These developments are promoting irreversible changes in the national health system and have thrown up several governance issues.

It is necessary to briefly mention the kind of shift that has taken place in the health policy profile consequent to the new direction of economy. Consistent with its market orientation, the new policy abandons its commitment to provide need-based free healthcare to all citizens. This implies that the citizens other than those who are officially recognized as 'poor' would have to pay for health services, except those relating to primary healthcare. The ambit of healthcare at the primary level itself has been restricted to preventive care, national disease control programmes and emergency services. The public health services are now required to generate resources to at least partly meet their cost of maintenance and expansion/improvement. Accordingly, user charges have been introduced in the public hospitals for non-poor seekers of healthcare. There is uninhibited commitment to promote the private sector (profit and non-profit) as an alternative mode of healthcare supply. The public sector healthcare is also required to trim its services and make way for private sector involvement by contracting out services to contain cost and achieve operational efficiency. The 'curative' healthcare is getting increasingly privatized since that is where the private sector is interested and its expansion is taking place. The expansion of public sector facilities is being confined to the difficult and inaccessible areas where the private sector, in any case, would not be interested to operate its services. The secondary and tertiary healthcare in the public sector is required, by and large, to become substantially self financing. Alternative modes of financing health services are being encouraged and promoted to lighten the responsibility of Government in provisioning of healthcare through measures such as public–private sector partnerships, health insurance, decentralized contributory healthcare arrangements, etc.

The major implication for health governance stems from the fact that the implementation of the new policy now requires less of government intervention and direct action in provisioning of health facilities but more of facilitation to permit other agencies to take up this task. The current dispensation requires administrative skills of persuasion and coordination rather than of planning and execution in health governance. This makes for a much lighter responsibility of the government, or rather, escape from it. The governance is now more riveted on enabling the private sector to supply health services, partner health development, share responsibility of the public sector healthcare, push in investment for expansion of facilities, engage in research and production of drugs, and set up institutions of medical education and training. The role of public sector healthcare now extends to outsourcing some of its activities, generating revenue to partly meet its cost, restructuring management of its existing services to achieve efficiency, improve quality and consumer satisfaction, effectively implementing programmes within its domain and arranging tie-ups with the private sector to make up for its management deficiencies. It was assumed that this lighter burden of health governance would improve the public sector healthcare by resolving issues carried over from the pre-reforms period. But the profile of health governance currently witnessed belies this assumption. Not only have the older governance issues lingered without being resolutely attended to, newer problems have emerged which pose an even greater challenge to the governability in health sector than what was experienced in the pre-reforms period.

Health Policy

Health sector reforms since the 1990s can be traced to three sources. One source was the macro-economic reforms mandated by the International Monetary Fund (IMF) as a part of the Structural Adjustment Programme (SAP). The second initiative came through health projects funded by the World Bank. The third source of reform flowed from the decision to integrate with the global economy. The SAP introduced fiscal discipline for stabilizing the economy which entailed curtailment of government expenditure. This inevitably led to the trimming of allocations in the social sector. The direct manifestation of this shift could be seen in reduced allocation for social services and welfare programmes, including health. The restructuring of economy also demanded, among others, curtailed ambit of public sector activities and liberalization of various sectors to make them competitive and market friendly. The reforms specific to the health sector were pursued by the World Bank as conditionalities to the projects financed by it. These included the disease control programmes of the Central government such as TB, leprosy, malaria, HIV-AIDS, blindness control and the state health systems projects at the state level whose focus was fixed on restructuring the secondary and tertiary level of healthcare. The nature of reforms pursued through this source has already been referred to. The participation in activities of the WTO and other global agencies of development entailed opening up of the health sector for trade, investment, research as well as implementation of the health programmes settled at the global level and collaboration with the multiple global institutions having interests in the health sector.

The impact of SAP could be felt in the dilution/loss of inter-sectoral support for attaining health outcomes (Qadeer, 2000) due to the reduced investment in social services (such as drinking water, sanitation, poverty alleviation and food security), diminished employment opportunities, low wages, difficult working conditions and environmental degradation. These developments affected the poor very adversely. The deceleration in capital expenditure on health led to stagnation in the health services. The health sector reforms introduced at the behest of the World Bank institutionalized a dual system of health services (under-funded public sector and well-funded and hi-tech private sector), access to which depended on the capacity of the service seeker to pay. The utility and utilization of primary healthcare was reduced due to non-availability of the health staff, investigative services and drugs, curtailed ambit of services and delinking of secondary and tertiary care from the primary healthcare. The externally aided health projects reinforced centralization and verticalization of the health programmes, introduced a techno-centric approach to their selection and prioritization, pushed technology choices and delivery systems overlooking the quality and spread of available infrastructure, social conditions of the majority population, and competence of the medical personnel. These projects unleashed new institutional arrangements which negatived the integrated approach to healthcare. This resulted in distorted investment pattern, weakening of state authority and political accountability and enormous problems of financial management, monitoring and coordination. The state health systems projects introduced dysfunctionalities in the public health system due to separate norms of expenditure, level of expenditure under different components unrelated to the specific local need, and institutional structures of programme management bypassing political control and involvement of the local democratic bodies (PRIs). The projects suffered from narrow focus, unsustainable expenditure, disproportionate drawl of financial and manpower resources from the existing public health system, absence of linkage with the central health programmes and failed to bridge inequities in the spread of health infrastructure between and within the states.

The reforms flowing from globalization are increasingly commodifying the health sector by stressing its potential for generating wealth. This radically changes its hitherto emphasized 'service' focus. The deregulation of health services and drug sector and its opening up for international trade and foreign direct investment have created different tiers of healthcare services in terms of cost, quality and use of technology, access to which is determined by the purchasing capacity of the patient. The promotion of medical tourism, export of manpower, corporatization of hospitals and outsourced clinical trials for drugs and devices have thrown up numerous adverse externalities. The global partnerships in health are laying down agenda of health programmes and use of technology therein for nations with no space of manoeuverability for them to escape from it. This is the perspective which informs governance of health emerging from the reforms.

Governance

The governance in the public health system in the post-reforms period would be examined with reference to two aspects: one, where the changes had impact on the users of health services and two, where the management of people's health was affected. The impact on users would be assessed in terms of instrumentality, functionality, access, cost, quality, equity of healthcare and its financing and regulation. The effect on the management of people's health would be evaluated in terms of the autonomy of decision making and the capacity to respond to the emerging threats to health of the people.

IMPACT ON USERS

Instrumentality

Mode of provisioning

The promotion of private sector healthcare has been actively pursued by the government through various policy instruments referred to earlier. These measures enabled the private sector to expand its activities and set up hi-tech healthcare facilities. Over the years, it has emerged as the dominant provider of curative healthcare. The health sector reforms have given a further fillip to this trend with the curtailment in expansion of the public sector healthcare units. The Tenth Five-Year Plan limits the establishment of public health facilities only to the exceptionally difficult and remote areas where the private sector has no interest in setting them up. The reforms have also encouraged outsourcing of certain services by the public hospitals to the private sector agencies and carving out a market for the private hospitals in curative services provided by the Government to its employees. The Government policy now vigorously advocates public-private partnerships as a new mode of provisioning services which imply sharing of tasks and responsibilities—financial, managerial and clinical in the public health system and setting up of new facilities to meet the national goals. The share of the Government in this partnership has taken various forms. The patterns of partnership include: (a) offering subsidized land, infrastructural development and equity participation for setting up tertiary and super specialty health facilities by the private sector, reduced interest on loans from public sector banks and fiscal concessions in the shape of reduced duties/exemptions for import of equipments by the private sector health units, (b) involving industry in managing the existing public health facilities with sharing of cost and responsibilities, (c) handing over management of the primary healthcare units in certain areas to the non-governmental and private sector organizations while continuing to meet their expenditure, (d) taking help of the private sector healthcare units in implementation of the national health programmes by obtaining specified services from them on payment, such as engaging the services of doctors/specialists against vacancies in rural health units, permitting them to carry out various components of a programme, (e) contracting out clinical and non-clinical services by the public hospitals to the private sector agencies, (f) hiring services of the doctors, specialists, para-medicos from the private health sector on contract basis, (g) reimbursing the private hospitals for specified procedures/ clinical treatment in respect of the patients registered with the Central government health scheme and the similar schemes of the PSUs. These partnerships have also extended to the setting up of joint ventures. A number of private hospitals have established collaborations with the public sector insurance corporations for providing services to their clients (Bhatt, 1993). This arrangement raises several governance issues. One of them relates to the questionable assumption of reformers about the perceived superiority of the private healthcare services in terms of cost efficiency and quality, which has not been empirically evaluated. The evidence has brought out that these partnerships have been introduced without adequate preparatory work such as regulatory instruments, monitoring arrangements, capacity building for financial analysis, legal scrutiny and negotiation ability, enforcement mechanism in respect of the terms of partnerships, specific assessment of how they would serve the policy goals of equity, efficiency, quality, etc. (Bhatt, 2000).

The consequences can be seen, for example, in the context of Delhi where the private hospitals, after availing of subsidy from the Government, have declined to honour the contractual obligation of providing free treatment to a specified number of poor patients. The Delhi government has failed to enforce the contract. A research study has highlighted a number of weaknesses in operating this arrangement in the cases studied. The evidence in this study brings out that the partnerships suffer from lack of a transparent policy frame, clarity on the terms of partnership, absence of focus on the consequences in terms of regional imbalance, unethical use of the facilities, demand inducement, cost escalation, practice of irrational medicine and techno interventions, dualism in standards of clinical care between the public and privately managed care, possible impact on the allocation of resources to the public sector healthcare, etc., which critically expose the incompetence of the government agencies in rushing through such proposals [Bhatt, 2000]. This has emerged as an altogether new governance issue not encountered in the pre-reforms period.

Financing of Healthcare

The most significant change that has taken place in the discourse on health policy in the post-reforms period is the shift in focus from provision of healthcare to financing of healthcare. The latter has acquired primacy in health planning and virtually relegated other issues of health governance to the background. This development is an offshoot of the new economic policies which are fixated on reducing public expenditure in provision of healthcare across the world. This objective was pursued by diversifying the mode of financing healthcare with a view to sharing the state's responsibility in providing health services. The modes of financing other than through public resources consist of the following options: Private sector (for profit), NGOs (non-profit), community organizations (through collective contribution), individuals (through contributory insurance/ direct purchase). The post-reforms period has seen efforts in promoting all these alternatives but, most conspicuously, private sector investment in provision of health services which the individuals, employers, companies (and, in some cases, state) can purchase. The NGO sector has also been encouraged to take up this role. But, given the lack of measurable success in mobilizing contribution from the members of the group catered to, the NGO alternative has not registered any significant presence. The community financing of healthcare has also faced a similar kind of problem. The share of the two, in any case, is very small. The individuals with assured purchasing power now extensively seek healthcare from the private healthcare providers. The contributory health insurance is confined to a small section of service seekers—the organized workers. It, however, meets only the hospitalization cost and excludes outpatient consultation for various illness episodes. In addition, the user charges for investigations and specified services in respect of outpatients and paying wards for inpatients have been introduced in the public hospitals to raise resources with the same objective of reducing the pressure on the Government to finance health services. This exercise in financing is designed to ensure that the entitlement to free healthcare is confined to preventive medicine, 'essential' primary care, disease control programmes and emergency services while the rest, particularly the curative care, is charged to the patient, except for people below poverty line. The discretionary illness fund and social insurance for which the premium is paid by the Government are alternative modes for meeting the health expenditure of persons below poverty line in respect of hospitalization. Apart from the iniquitous access to healthcare involved in this arrangement, these interventions have not reduced the dependence of a large section of the population on public-funded healthcare, given their inability to purchase healthcare from the private sector health facilities or contribute towards accessing it in NGO or community-administered health facility. The attempts at garnering resources by the public hospitals through levy of user charges and introduction of private wards have failed to generate sufficient amount to reduce responsibility of the Government for meeting their resource requirements. Since the level of public expenditure on health as a percentage of GDP (0.9%) is among the lowest in the world, these changes have had the effect of reducing access of the poorer sections to healthcare, increasing indebtedness of those who sought healthcare from the market despite its un-affordability, forcing the very poor to avoid seeking healthcare altogether and producing overall adverse health outcomes for these sections. The situation that emerged as a result of these changes underlines sharply the need for strengthening public-funded services and enhancing public expenditure on health for this purpose.

In the circumstances, increasing public health expenditure as the desirable mode of financing healthcare emerges as a major issue. The governance discourse has dealt with three modes of stepping up state's contribution to healthcare services: tax revenue, external finance and user charges. The third alternative holds no promise, as the experience of low realization has shown. In any case, the user charges constitute contribution of the patients and not of the state and the meagre resources so generated carry a huge social cost. The option of external finance is being increasingly relied upon. But this mode of financing restricts the autonomy of use and is unsustainable besides creating distortions in the optimum use of available public resources. Yet, it continues to be the preferred mode for financing programmes considered 'essential' by the donor agencies. The alternative of generating additional tax revenues for this purpose has not been sufficiently explored. The reluctance to enhance the level of taxation from the richer sections is on account of its perceived adverse impact on investment climate in the neo-liberal economy adopted by the country. The health governance has, therefore, to resolve the conflict between two objectives of the state policy: one of encouraging private investment for boosting growth and the other of ensuring equitable access to comprehensive healthcare to improve health outcomes and, therefore, to adopt sustainable means to meet public expenditure for this purpose.

Functionality

One of the recurring complaints in the pre-reforms period affecting the functionality of health services related to the non-availability of health personnel and drugs. The impact of reforms on this problem can now be assessed.

Health manpower

The public health system right from inception has suffered from non-availability of the doctors/specialists and para-medical personnel in the healthcare units located in the rural areas. In the early years of Independence, it may have been on account of insufficient number of available trained graduates/ postgraduates against the spurt of demand in the primary healthcare facilities which were being set up in the rural areas.

But over the years, the medical education infrastructure has expanded and, in the post-reforms period, private medical colleges have mushroomed, particularly in the southern states. With an admission capacity exceeding 17,000 graduates in 405 colleges, there is one doctor for 1500 persons and, if ISM & H doctors are included, one for 800. Yet, the staff shortage exists to the extent of 15 – 20% in the cities but is more severe in the rural areas. This has occurred due to out-migration besides disinclination of the medical professionals to work in the rural areas. The brain drain has been acute in the super specialty institutions like AIIMS (Delhi) and PGI (Chandigarh). The Government has been disinclined to check this flight of talent despite the huge public funds spent on their training. This issue was raised by many critics in the pre-reforms period but there was little by way of checkmating migration due to the enormous clout of doctors. The trend has increased in the post-reforms period with the globalization of economy and the relative ease of manpower movement across nations. Still worse, under GATS (WTO, 1995), the Government itself is vigorously pursuing liberalization of international trade regime for movement of manpower across countries under mode 4 of the agreement and advocating relaxation of immigration and other regulatory arrangements introduced by the developed countries for this purpose.

The brain drain in health manpower is not confined to the doctors and specialists but extends to the nurses and other paramedics (physiotherapists, technicians handling hi-tech equipments, for example). There is a growing demand for them both in the developed and the developing countries. In fact, powerful advocacy is at work for the medical education curricula to be tailored to international specifications and demand with a view to satisfying the requirements for export of health manpower. A more disturbing development is that the corporate sector hospitals within the country are also poaching on the doctors, specialists and paramedics working in the public sector hospitals with attractive financial benefits. This has led to many senior specialists in the public hospitals leaving their jobs to join the private sector health facilities. The private sector healthcare, thus, gets highly skilled and experienced health manpower without any cost while the public healthcare finds it difficult to fill the slots vacated by such migration. Medical tourism is intensifying this development of internal brain drain as the best trained personnel go over to the institutions that cater to the foreign patients (JSA, 2009). This amounts to a virtual subsidization of the foreign patients. In the coming years, both these trends would increase. This would have a debilitating effect on the functioning of the public health system and would also lead to distortions in the content of medical education to suit the pattern of demand in national and international market. The objective of training doctors to work in the rural areas would be virtually impossible to achieve, notwithstanding the promise made in the National Rural Health Mission document that it would be pursued vigorously. The governance in the health sector is faced with the complex task of resolving the conflict between the growth imperative of economy as also the values and aspirations of medical professionals and the needs of healthcare of the rural areas.

Availability of Drugs

The low access to drugs on account of poverty is already a serious problem in the healthcare profile of the country. The population that can access essential drugs ranges between 20 and 40% (JSA, 2009). The inadequate supply of drugs in the public health system is a major reason for its under-utilization by the poorer sections (Bhargava et al., 2006). The expenditure on drugs in medicare is an important cause of indebtedness in the rural areas. In the pre-reforms period, the Government was faced with serious problems posed by the pattern of manufacture, distribution and pricing of drugs due to the dominance of the private sector (MNCs) in this industry. It made efforts to restructure this arrangement but did not succeed in this objective because of the enormous power enjoyed by the foreign drug companies. The drug scene currently is characterized by shortage of essential drugs, but excess of costly, hazardous and irrational drugs besides sub standard, spurious and even banned drugs floating in the market (Shiva, et al., 2004). The drug production is distorted in favour of irrational and expensive drugs with nearly 40,000 formulations and numerous brands of the same in circulation (VHAI, 1997). As per the current estimate, more than 80,000 brands are marketed in India (JSA, 2009). The prescription behaviour of treating healthcare professionals is influenced by aggressive salesman-ship of the manufacturing drug companies and incentives given to them while the distribution is guided by hefty trade margins. The drug prices show enormous variation in retail, going up sometimes to more than 1000% (Locost, 2004; Bhargava et al., 2006). The essential drugs are increasingly becoming out of reach for the majority of the Indian population.

In the pre-reforms period, while the structural issues relating to drug industry could not be addressed, the Government mitigated the difficulties faced by consumers to some extent by two measures, which sought to make essential drugs available at affordable prices. The one consisted of taking up production of some essential drugs in the public sector and the other comprised introducing price control which applied to 342 drugs as per the Drug Price Control Order, 1979. The economic reforms have undone both these measures. The public sector production has collapsed, running up huge losses. In addition, the new Pharmaceutical Policy (2002) has deregulated the drug industry removing all protection provided to the public sector units earlier (MoC, 2002). Recently, the public sector vaccine-producing units have also been closed down (Raghuram, 2008). The Drug Price Control Order has reduced the number of drugs to 73 in 2003 (this decision has been challenged in the Supreme Court). There is a palpable resistance to impose price control on essential drugs due to which even the limited control resorted to has become ineffective (JSA, 2009). These developments have led to the rise in prices of essential drugs. The complexity of governance in this matter is reflected in the conflict between the goals pursued by two sectors of development—industry and health. The Pharmaceutical Policy 2002 is focused on the growth of industry and encouragement of private sector investment rather than on ensuring availability of essential drugs at affordable prices to the people and, therefore, is in conflict with the National Health Policy 2002 which promotes people's access to cheaper drugs for improving health outcomes.

Yet another complexity has been added. The TRIPS regime of international trade has made patented drugs even more expensive than other drugs. The amendment to the Indian Patent Act in 2005 has foreclosed the option of producing generic substitutes of these drugs by alternative processes. Therefore, the cost of new drugs patented by MNCs as also new life-saving drugs needed for treatment of HIV-AIDS, cancer, etc. is prohibitive and, therefore, unaffordable to most people in the country. The MNCs use their clout and resources to prevent national production of these drugs permissible under the TRIPS agreement through issuance of compulsory licenses. The issue was pursued at the global level through the collective efforts of the adversely affected developing countries and some success was achieved in respect of the drugs used for treatment of HIV-AIDS. But this concession is inadequate to address the huge adverse impact of new patent regime on availability of patented life-saving drugs.

The enforcement of regulations in the field of drugs is another area of concern where the deficit of governance has attracted the attention of the Supreme Court too. The regulatory regime relating to drugs suffers from weak laws, inadequate personnel for inspection, investigation and filing prosecution and dismal record of securing convictions. This has made the task of checking the sale of spurious and hazardous drugs and circulation of banned drugs enormously difficult, which led the Supreme Court to intervene in the matter. The Mashelkar Committee set up by the Government in this context has given a number of recommendations which have formed the basis of the proposed amendments to the existing law. No changes in regulations have been effected so far.

The promotion of competition by deregulation of drug industry has not led to cheaper drugs being available as the drug prices in the country are supplier driven, with little consumer awareness and resistance. In the circumstances, making drugs available to the people at affordable prices has emerged as an even more challenging governance issue in the current economy than it was in the pre-reforms period. On the other hand, the Government has lesser autonomy and also lesser inclination to control drug industry in the post-reforms period than it ever had in the pre-reforms period. The recently proposed inclusion of a larger number of drugs under the Drug Price Control Order under pressure of a pending PIL in the Supreme Court has met with strong resistance from the industry. It is not certain whether even this limited intervention would materialize.

Access to healthcare

In view of the differential level of entitlements and available services, there are huge problems in accessing need-based healthcare, particularly by those sections who do not have the necessary purchasing power. This problem extends to accessing public sector healthcare where user charges and paying wards have been introduced for revenue generation. The section of population that is facing stress on this account is quite large and is also differentiated within itself in terms of the levels of income and social conditions. The Government has responded to this problem by exempting 'BPL' (Below Poverty Line) patients from payment of user charges in the public hospitals. But this limited concession ignores the social realities. First, even this 'exemption' or 'free treatment' for BPL patients camouflages the restrictions placed on this entitlement. It does not cover all expenditure of treatment. The BPL patient would have to incur considerable out of pocket expenditure in the case of hospitalization. This deficiency is sought to be met by providing needy patients financial grants from special funds (National Illness Assistance Fund at the central level or the National Relief Fund where the PM has some discretion) or similar discretionary funds, if existing at the state level. This arrangement for meeting the cost of hospitalization, however, is not available in many states. Even where it exists, its small corpus cannot meet the gigantic problem of disbursing the cost of hospitalization incurred by the poor people whose number is very large. Besides, even after availing of this assistance, the residual expenditure would still have to be met by the patient. The latest response of the Government is to provide social insurance. A scheme called the Rashtriya Bima Yojana has been launched, which would provide Rs. 30,000 in patient health benefit at a premium of Rs. 600 which the Government would pay in the case of BPL persons (Das, 2008). Notwithstanding the fact that a patient can choose from a list of private and public hospitals for treatment under the scheme, there are too many uncertainties and operational difficulties in availing of any social health insurance by the poor (Garg, 2006). Second, the admissibility of exemption from payment of user charges or any other such concession is conditional upon the patient's producing a BPL certificate. This certificate is not easy to obtain because of the problems associated with the process of identification of BPL persons and preparation of the BPL list. The difficulties in negotiating with the bureaucracy to obtain a BPL certificate would, therefore, exclude many deserving persons from accessing the benefits of exemption from user charges in the case of OPD services and the cost of treatment in the case of in-patient hospitalisation. It would also stand in the way of obtaining the benefit of health insurance if such a certificate is insisted upon. The more serious problem, however, is that the officially prepared BPL list excludes a large number of poor who cannot afford to purchase healthcare. As of now, they have no entitlement to exemption. These persons would either have to borrow and become indebted in seeking healthcare or ignore their illness and avoid medical consultation altogether. Both options have adverse implications for health outcomes of the country.

The practice of user charges in public health facilities is also changing the orientation of service providers. The managements in these hospitals seek to attract paying patients rather than expand and improve the facilities for poorer patients. The levy of user charges over a period of time also impacts on the quality of services extended to the two segments of patients—the paying and the non-paying. It, in fact, subsidizes the better-off sections (paying patients) as more resources are directed to meet their needs. Besides, the collections from user charges even after periodic revisions are too small to even partly substitute for government funding of the concerned public health institutions (Baru, 2001) which puts a question mark on the rationale and utility of this measure. In the context of depressing health indicators, ensuring access to need-based healthcare for all those who cannot afford to pay is a huge challenge to governance that has been posed in the post-reforms phase. Sustaining the 'service' orientation of public health institutions and extending uniform quality of services by its providers unrelated to the paying capacity is the other demanding task.

Cost of healthcare

The rising cost of healthcare is a serious barrier to access services for a large section of the population, leaving aside a small percentage of the affluent persons. The cost of healthcare has enormously increased with the expansion of private sector facilities and, in particular, the entry of the corporate and foreign investors in this sector. The assumption that market forces through competition would bring down the cost has been totally belied. Healthcare is a supply-driven service. The excessive use of hi-tech in private sector healthcare is driving the cost of treatment higher. This facet has emerged from policy instruments which subsidized the cost of equipments imported by the private hospitals. Medical tourism is further fuelling this trend. There is no regulatory body at present to evaluate the merits of technology used in healthcare in terms of the utility, safety and cost before its introduction in the health system. The hi-tech bias in private healthcare also generates pressures on the public health system to follow suit. The irrational medicine practised through unnecessary investigations and expensive drugs is yet another factor contributing to the cost escalation. For all these reasons, the expenditure on medicare is increasing and has emerged as the second largest cause of indebtedness in the country. It affects not only the poor but the middle class as well. More than one-third of such persons slide below the poverty line as a result of meeting the cost of hospitalization. The out-of-pocket expenditure pushes 2.2% of the population below poverty line in one year (Mishra et al., 2003). Lowering the cost of healthcare and cutting down the use of hi-tech equipments, unnecessary investigations and expensive drugs in its practice is a major governance problem waiting to be tackled. This is largely a post-reforms issue.

Quality of healthcare

In the pre-reforms period, the discourse on quality of healthcare was focused largely on the public health facilities in view of their dominant position. The issues of quality were raised, by and large, in the context of primary healthcare due to its non-functional character—absence of doctors, non-availability of drugs, ill-equipped physical and investigative infrastructure and poor maintenance of facilities. The indifferent and unhelpful behaviour of service providers was another sore point. The quality of secondary and tertiary health was also compromised by long queues, over-crowding, non-functional equipments, inadequate funds for maintenance, drugs, lack of sufficient attention from the treating doctors, etc. The post-reforms discourse has thrown up huge problems of quality, both in public and private sector healthcare. The quality and management of healthcare in the private hospitals has come in for scathing attack in respect of all conceivable parameters—high cost, unnecessary investigations, practice of irrational medicine, negligence, incompetence of service providers, unethical practices, violations of municipal laws, etc. The service seekers also find that there is no credible functioning mechanism to check the quality of care and standards of treatment by which the responsibility of providers can be pinned down for holding them accountable for lapses. The regulatory bodies—the medical councils—provide no relief and even recourse to judicial courts leads to frustration. The public healthcare has also failed to set up standards to be emulated by the private sector. The complaints of patients in public hospitals are increasing. Overcrowding, long waiting queues, inadequate capacity, indifferent service, non-functioning equipments, insensitive behaviour of doctors and paramedical staff and negligence in treatment continue to be reported in the public health services. The pressure of number of patients on the one hand and resource crunch on the other contribute considerably to the poor quality of care in the public health units. But it is equally true that the transparent mechanisms of providing quality assurance and enforcing quality control are also absent in public sector facilities. There are no protocols of standards for facilities, services and treatment in the public health system against which the patients or their relatives can evaluate the quality of services received and no credible arrangement of grievance redressal which the persons with complaints can approach for getting relief. In the post-reforms period, the deficiencies of quality in healthcare have exacerbated due to the dual service regime—one for the paying patients and the other for the non-paying ones, the former getting better services than the latter. The absence of continuing education of healthcare providers particularly those in the rural healthcare also impacts on the quality of services they render. The professional self-regulatory mechanisms have failed to work. This applies both to the western medicine as well as the Indian systems of medicine and homoeopathy.

The problems of quality are shocking in respect of the unqualified private practitioners whose number is almost equal to the qualified ones and who cater to the poorest sections in view of the low cost of their treatment and the ease with which they can be accessed. Their medicare practice is illegal but they fill a huge gap in access created by the public and private (qualified) health services. The poor enforcement of law and absence of alternative for patients have sustained this arrangement, which carries enormous risk to the life and health of the patients accessing these services. The healthcare provided by the NGOs and the traditional healthcare workers also remains outside the ambit of regulation and, therefore, there is no assurance of quality in the services they provide.

The most important governance issue in respect of the quality of healthcare, both in the public and the private health facilities, relates to setting up of effective and credible regulatory arrangements and a transparent mechanism of redressal of complaints which inspire public confidence and enforce accountability of health staff involved. In addition, adequate provision of funds would be required to improve the quality of public health services. A system of compulsory and periodic training of the healthcare practitioners in the rural health care is necessary in respect of both. The pattern of health manpower production also needs to be drastically changed to ensure availability of the doctors/specialists in the under-served areas. All these issues have figured in the discourse on post-reforms health governance.

Regulation

The absence of regulation was felt even during the pre-reforms period when the public health sector was a major provider of services and the private sector was beginning to grow from the mid-1980s. But a pronounced trend towards privatization of curative healthcare that has come up with the reforms has brought out the deficit of regulation glaringly.

The areas needing regulations have enormously widened while the response of the Government in providing them is in inverse proportion. The huge expansion of the private sector healthcare with frequent incidents of negligence, irrational treatment, unnecessary procedures and investigations calls for swift action to protect healthcare seekers. The entry of MNCs in the health sector with cross-national dimensions of their operations underlines the need for widening the range of regulations to deal with the complexity involved. The unabated surge in the use of hi-technology in healthcare would call for a mechanism to evaluate its need, cost and effect on people's health as well as regulation of its use. Medical tourism also needs to be checked for its fallout in terms of sucking poor people into organ donation, hosting of surrogate pregnancy, etc. The BPOs in medical research need to be mandatorily registered, stringently screened and effectively monitored to protect the poor and gullible patients from suffering the consequences of being used as subjects of clinical trials with serious risks to their life and health. The incidence of adulteration in articles of consumption has enormously increased and now extends to a larger number of commodities in common use, signifying infirmities in law, and poor investigation and prosecuting abilities. The public–private partnerships have exposed the absence of regulation to hold the private partner accountable for its obligation and to protect public partner's interests. A large number of healthcare providers operate informally and are outside the ambit of any regulation. All such health workers need to be covered by regulations including those who would now be working under the NRHM. The operations of the drug sector have multi-faceted impact on people's lives. This sector calls for a comprehensive and stringent regulatory arrangement beyond the existing ones. The free flow of goods under the new regime of international trade is introducing new products of consumption, many of which could pose grave risks to the health and lives of people. This area has not even been mapped out, let alone regulated. The microbial unification of the world has exposed our people and livestock to new diseases and risks of infection. Our regulatory arrangements to check their entry and manage the fallout are outmoded and require a comprehensive revision.

The agenda, evidently, is large as we seriously lag behind in terms of health regulations. As for the enforcement of existing regulations, the position is worse. This is due to the deficiencies in respect of personnel, investigative facilities, prosecuting ability, training, monitoring arrangements and allocation of resources. It is evident that the health laws are in need of extensive overhaul, as would appear from the poor enforcement in checking fraudulent kidney donations and sale of spurious substandard and hazardous drugs (Menon, 2002). The capacity for enforcement of health laws requires considerable upgradation in terms of additional personnel, intensive training, higher allocation, augmentation of investigative infrastructure and result-oriented monitoring. The proliferation of substandard medical training institutions with inadequate teaching faculty and absence of essential infrastructure has already exposed the fragility of the existing regulatory provisions. The existing regulations would, therefore, need to be tightened and made more stringent and the new laws would have to be enacted or provisions added to the existing laws to adequately cover the emerging areas of health hazards. There is no greater pointer to the deficit of governance in this area than the fact that the initiative for strengthening health laws and their implementation has come from the apex court rather than the Government itself.

Equity in Healthcare

The paradigm of development lays down not only policies and instruments for creation of wealth through economic growth but also mechanisms for distribution of resources so generated among social groups claiming a share or needing help. This distributive dimension has overriding implications for promoting social justice because it creates stakes for various social groups in the development process. In the health sub-sector of social development, more than in any other sub-sector, distributive aspects have great significance because health policies and programmes tend to affect individuals and social groups differentially. If the programme benefits are skewedly distributed, adverse health outcomes for a large section of population may be the consequence. This may, in turn, affect not only the economy and productivity but also the overall health of society. In the pre-reforms period, equitable distribution of income and social benefits was accepted as a goal to be pursued, though the seriousness of its pursuit by the Government could be questioned. Accordingly, a variety of programme interventions such as those relating to poverty reduction, subsidized social services, welfare measures were made to reduce inequalities and improve the economic status of poorer and marginalized sections. With the onset of economic reforms, this goal of equity has taken a backseat though some of the pre-reform programmes continue to operate. In the changed development paradigm, inequities resulting from economic growth have increased manifold but the urge to bridge them has evaporated. In fact, the growth itself is perceived by policy makers to reduce inequities in the long run. The inequities are thus considered inevitable and conducive to progress.

In the health sub-sector, despite commitment to provide affordable healthcare to all sections of the population, serious inequities have emerged in the access to healthcare, utilization of health facilities and quality of services rendered. These inequities are multi-dimensional. These are reflected in the sharp rural-urban differentials in availability of health facilities and quality of care they extend. Disparities also exist in availability of facilities across states, some providing better and more dispersed facilities than others. This skewness also exists between developed and backward regions/districts within states. This dimension of inequity points towards geographical disparity in distribution.

There are also inequities in access to healthcare facilities influenced by economic as well as social status. This is manifested in the lower access of SCs, STs and Muslim minority to services provided therein as against upper-caste Hindus. The reduced access of women to health services is another dimension of the iniquitous access to healthcare. The income-based disparities are significantly indicated by the degree of access to healthcare facilities and the extent of services utilized by the poorer sections as compared to the better-off groups.

The inequities can also be observed, and very sharply, in the quality of healthcare extended by the facilities and service providers. The urban areas and developed regions offer more comprehensive care and of better quality as the health care units have doctors/specialists/para-medics in position and are equipped with better investigative facilities and physical infrastructure. The rural health facilities suffer from absence of doctors/para-medics, non-functioning equipments, poor infrastructure and non supply of drugs. This differential in quality of care is also a function of differential resource distribution—financial and manpower—in the two regions. The inequities also extend to skewed access to information and health education, both between geographical areas as well as among social groups.

These inequities are faithfully manifested in the differential health outcomes among social groups. The poorer sections as against richer brackets, SCs/STs in comparison to upper castes, Muslims in contrast to Hindus, women as against men in each social segment have a lower (adverse) attainments in respect of various indicators of good health. They have lower level of access to and utilization of health services but make higher level of out-of-pocket expenditure on health.

These inequities existed in the pre-reforms period as well despite the commitment of the Government to reduce them and a host of welfare programmes contributing towards this effort. The economic and health sector reforms have widened these inequities. The available data from NSSO surveys in 1986–1996 together with other empirical studies suggest worsening of class-based inequalities in access to health services. This can be seen in conjunction with the decline in utilization of out-patient services by the proportion of patients in public hospitals from 17.7 to 11% of the total in the rural areas and from 22.6 to 15% in the urban areas. The public hospitals were used more by the better-off in the 1990s than the poorer groups. With the sharp decline in total rural hospitalization rates from 60 to 44%, the implication is that the poor are not able to access health services. As a consequence, the untreated morbidity among the lower most fractile increased to 39% in rural and 61% in urban areas between these periods. The number of those who cited financial reasons for the inability to access healthcare went up from 15 to 24% in the rural areas and from 10 to 21% in the urban areas (Sen et al., 2002). There would be little doubt that socially excluded groups would form a larger portion of those who could not access health services on grounds of income. But inequities are also caused by accessing healthcare with borrowed resources due to insufficient purchasing power. The expenditure on healthcare has emerged as one of the most important causes of indebtedness and contributes to the increasing poverty. Forty per cent of the hospitalized people are forced to borrow money or sell assets to cover expenses. More than two crore people slide below the poverty line due to out-of-pocket expenditure on healthcare (JSA, 2009). This leads to the lowering of economic status which, in turn, reduces access to healthcare in future.

The economic class-based inequities have also widened with the expansion of private sector healthcare units and the state-of-art corporate hospitals. The increasing cost of healthcare has created different layers of access determined by the levels of purchasing power. The rural and urban differentials in healthcare facilities have further increased as the private sector expansion has taken place in the urban areas and prosperous rural pockets. The non-functionality of primary healthcare facilities shows no sign of improvement in terms of attendance of doctors and availability of drugs. With the onset of TRIPS and a new patent law on the statute book, the prices of patented drugs have increased. With reduced number of drugs under the Drug Price Control Order, even the non-patented drugs are becoming out of reach for the poorer people more than they were earlier.

These inequities in healthcare are the outcome of multiple factors. Reducing them would imply addressing all the factors—availability, functionality, access, cost, quality, financial allocation, human resource management, etc. These problems along with their suggested solutions have been a part of health governance discourse for a long time. The recently launched NRHM is a belated attempt to deal with some of them. The nature of interventions made to address them and the degree of success achieved in this effort would reflect on the governance ability of decision makers and their seriousness to pursue equity goals.

Management of People's Health

Autonomy in decision making

No single factor has affected the policy and governance in the health sector so much as the external influence exercised by the aid and lending (donor) agencies. It is, therefore, necessary to analytically present in some detail the nature of their intervention and its impact on the public health system.

The externally-aided projects in general are considered to have a damaging effect on internal national planning because of their shorter mission, narrow focus, emphasis on operational rather than strategic aspects and unsustainability in terms of building local capacity (Green, 1995). In India, the Government has been accepting external assistance for health programmes since independence. While the share of external funding constitutes only 1–3% of the government expenditure on health

[Mishra et al., 2003], it has exercised influence on the health policy and governance disproportionate to this meagre contribution. The external projects have distorted national priorities and reduced accountability of the government (Chatterjee, 1988; Baru and Jessani, 2000) In the pre-reforms period, malaria and leprosy programmes and medical education were major areas of assistance in the early years (Jeffrey, 1988). The subsequent funding largely concentrated on Family Planning including Maternal and Child Health (MCH), immunization, primary healthcare for strengthening delivery of services and upgrading skills of the implementing personnel. In the 1990s, the size of assistance increased and the emphasis shifted to sectoral policy interventions. In the early years, the pattern of external assistance was grants-in-aid for specific programmes. The donors were bilateral agencies largely. The World Bank has emerged on the scene since the 1980s as a major provider of assistance for population stabilization projects of the Government. The economic reforms paved the way for a larger thrust of external assistance starting with HIV-AIDS and, thereafter, extending to malaria, TB, leprosy, blindness control besides Reproductive and Child Health (RCH). Later, 'state health systems' projects were also taken up for assistance exclusively focusing on secondary healthcare. This expansion was directly related to the amenability of policy establishment to accept policy changes in the health sector.

The project mode was the pattern of this assistance by the World Bank and bilateral agencies, by and large. These projects were focused on the specific programmes and carried conditionalities which had to be rigorously adhered to. The experience of implementation of these projects has brought out certain features of this mode of assistance which impinge on health governance. These features, in brief, are:

- Exclusivity in terms of attention, management, financing, norms and procedures of expenditure and reporting
- Centralization, verticalization and bureaucratization of the organizational structure and decision-making process

- Creation of new management structures—a hierarchy of implementing/delivery agencies
- Strict adherence to the approved design of the project with little autonomy to deviate from the directions; excessive emphasis on reporting, monitoring and inspections
- Engagement of a battery of consultants, foreign and Indian, disregarding local/internal expertise
- 'Stand alone' character of the projects with no linkages to the other programmes
- Resort to global tendering for procurement of commodities, construction activities and provision of services
- Enforcement of the segmented and rigid distribution of funds, activity wise with no flexibility to implementing agencies
- Drawing of human and financial resources from other programmes/activities in the public health sector
- Creating an adverse impact on the health programmes not funded externally
- Un-sustainability in terms of durability, financing and quality

These externally-aided projects carried three sets of conditionalities. One related to the acceptance of policy frame which included the content of technical direction. This involved consenting to the technology for investigation, treatment regimen and operational research, associating private sector in implementation, introducing cost containment measures, etc. The second set of conditionalities related to the institutional control covering delivery system, norms of resource utilization and monitoring arrangement. The third set of conditionalities envisaged separate management structures for efficient decision making bypassing the existing decision making process in the health organization. These conditionalities created several problems. In respect of the disease control programmes, these requirements restricted the selection process to diseases where technology-based intervention could yield effective results instead of conventional epidemiological basis, social dimensions of disease and the range of coverage for prioritization of health intervention. The organizational approach distorted the investment pattern and disregarded the horizontal arrangement of delivery in the primary health care. The projects also promoted greater centralization in health planning and implementation and, thus, weakened the autonomy of the state agencies to tackle health problems. The management structures, in particular, created dysfunctionalities in the working of public health system by creating duality of norms and procedures for undertaking expenditure, drawing of personnel and resources from other programmes and bypassing existing arrangements of decision making and political control. The level of resources committed to the projects created problems of durability and sustainability as well.

That these conditionalities were accepted while negotiating the projects showed the degree of pressure exerted by the funding agencies and the inability of the concerned central and state officials to stand up to them. The degree of reverence shown to the lending agencies in this matter lays bare the weaknesses of the bureaucracy and the over zealousness of the central and state governments to get the projects sanctioned at all costs ignoring the long-term consequences. This lack of capacity or will to resist pressures is a failing which is waiting to be recognized as a governance problem. In the post-reforms period, the World Bank officials loom large over the health policy establishment. The authority which these officials manage to exercise and the consideration that is shown to them even by the highest functionaries of the Government has implications for the autonomy of state to design a health policy and evolve institutional arrangements for delivery suited to its people. This aspect of governance creates particular unease at a time when political direction in the matter is virtually non-existent.

Capacity to intervene

The working of the health sector has exposed a serious lack of capacity to govern. This has been evident in the pre-reforms phase itself. The vision of health outlined in the policy design after Independence was embedded in its 'developmental' dimension. This implied that the health governance should create conditions in which people can stay healthy. To effectuate this goal, appropriate integration of social determinants of health with healthcare arrangement was necessary. This objective, however, remained unrealized due to, among others, the incapacity of health bureaucracy to creatively coordinate with other agencies implementing social sector programmes which had a bearing on the health of the people. In the post-reforms phase, the market is assumed to replace the state in promoting good health. The market obviously cannot discharge this function. The critical issue of governance is how public policy in sectors other than health should be influenced to obtain favourable health outcomes. This requires two things. First, it should be ensured that promoting good health should become central to the political agenda of the country. Second, the state's health agency should have the capacity to assess the impact of policies and governance in other sectors on the health of the people (Lavis and Sullivan, 1999). Neither of the two things happen at present. To create the necessary political will for promoting people's health, relevant information needs to be collected on the impact of sectoral activities on health and the analysis based on it to be placed before the political decision makers. The nodal health governance agency does not seem to undertake this exercise in any systemic and sustained manner. The new economic policies have adversely impacted the social constituents of health in diverse ways. The upswing of economic growth has not kept pace with creation of employment and alleviation of poverty. The wage levels and working conditions for a large section of the people have sharply deteriorated. The provisioning of subsidized social services is under threat of shrinkage, if not elimination altogether. The degradation of environment, destabilization/loss of livelihoods, large scale displacement from land, habitat and income-earning avenues, increased migration with unhealthy living conditions, exposure to hazardous technology, informalization of work, rising incidence of child labour and trafficking of women and children have implications for the health of population. The disturbing effects of international trade on changes in diets, induced consumption of products injurious to health, contaminated food products, dumping of hazardous technologies, proliferation of toxic waste in the living environment, all pose serious threats to the people's health. The aggressive consumerism and import of cultural products are promoting an unhealthy lifestyle and disintegrating the social support system which increase mental disorders and suicides. The microbial traffic through increased human contact is giving rise to new diseases. Greater priority and enhanced capacity is needed to promote social conditions for good health than what was required in the pre-reforms phase. Yet, ironically, the subject occupies much less space in the political agenda of the country. There is a glaring lack of capacity in the state health agencies to link the existing public policies with deteriorating health of the people and prepare material evidence in this regard both for advocacy and corrective intervention. Creating this capacity in health agencies to analyze health implications of the current paradigm of economic growth and to use this evidence to create necessary political will to neutralize the adverse externalities is a governance issue which cannot be overemphasized.

This capacity 'deficit' also emanates from lack of jurisdiction of the organization dealing with the health policy in the government (central or state) in respect of sectoral activities which create ill health—trade, industry, agriculture, mining, urban development, labour as well as fiscal and monetary policies. The sectoral activities are distributed in different ministries with each exercising exclusive bureaucratic and political control in its domain. The 'horizontal fragmentation' (Lavis and Sullivan, 1999) in governance structures prevents coordinated action in this regard. Each sectoral agency focuses on its exclusive interests and ignores or minimizes externalities on health in the pursuit of its growth. The Planning Commission as the overarching development outfit could discharge the role of taking a larger view of sectoral development to check adverse health outcomes. But it neither has the political clout nor the capacity to do so. Creating this capacity, therefore, would call for a specific mandate in the rules of business of the Government, input of resources—financial, man power and training, and setting up of an institutional mechanism within the Government to deal with inter-sectoral conflicts emerging from the investigations of the nodal health agency, civil society organizations and institutions of social science research. Lest an intra-government body minimize the adverse externalities of economic growth on people's health, a cross-sectoral/non-official autonomous body outside the Government would need to be promoted, in addition, to create pressures on the Government and raise public debate on this issue.

The capacity deficit also relates to another emerging area of concern. This lies in the expanding area of trade negotiations and other global interactions. There are health implications of several proposals discussed therein which are never taken into account due to lack of knowledge in the negotiators who happen to be trade or sector-specific officials. Even the Ministry of Health has no built-in capacity to comprehensively examine such proposals and provide policy briefs to the negotiating team except where it is specifically consulted on a subject directly concerning health. The result is that once agreements are concluded, there is no way to disregard them if adverse externalities emerge. There is, therefore, a need to create this capacity in the Ministry of Health to furnish policy briefs and, where necessary, associate health officials during the course of negotiations.

The capacity deficit has another dimension which has been inherited from the pre-reforms period. This involves convergence of health programmes with those in other social sectors which have a positive impact on promoting good health both at the policy making as well as the implementation level. The distinguishing feature here is that there is no conflict of interests between the sectoral agencies and the health organization. The weakness lies in lack of a focused institutional mechanism for such deliberations, absence of vigorous interaction between agencies dealing with health and other development sectors and efforts to forge convergence. Currently, each sectoral organization monitors and evaluates its programmes in terms of goals it has set in respect of them but does not relate them to the impact on health of the beneficiaries

(Chatterjee, 1988). Though a broad positive externality for health is perceived while formulating and sanctioning individual programmes, this is not sufficient for articulating with sufficient clarity what health goals are sought to be achieved and how each programme would contribute towards them with specific reference to the targeted areas and social groups. It, therefore, becomes necessary for the nodal health agency to define its goals, identify which deficiencies constrain their realization and in which sectoral jurisdiction they lie and how the programme/ programmes taken up by the concerned agencies would neutralize these constraints. This function cannot be discharged merely by the routine consultation process which takes place at present. The convergence actually does not get effected at any level in the Government—central, state, district or panchayat. The policy makers complacently feel that convergence will get effected by itself or by issue of instructions. This will not happen without a proper institutional mechanism and focused efforts dedicated to it. The capacity creation here would require the nodal health organization to identify goals requiring cross-sectoral development support, produce relevant profile of the targeted areas and population groups where these goals have to be pursued, and pass on the information to the concerned sectoral agency for appropriate integration. The Planning Commission has to ensure at the time of approval of sectoral plans and programmes that specific linkages are created and embedded in the Plan document along with the mechanism of convergence and monitoring. Thereafter, the nodal health agency has to work out state, district, panchayat-wise details with the help of state governments, tie up the loose ends and develop indicators by which the impact will be monitored. This does not happen at present. The nodal health agency has no capacity or urge to discharge this responsibility nor have the sectoral programme agencies taken initiative to forge these linkages. To create the will to pursue this objective and the capacity to translate it into tangible action is the task of governance. But, in doing so, bottlenecks may emerge to stall such convergence caused by the rigid schematic structures and guidelines of the programmes, mechanisms of implementation or objections of the funding agencies. The nodal health organization has to identify such bottlenecks and get them sorted out at the inter-agency decision making levels failing which at the level of the cabinet. The governance dimension of this issue lies in the capacity building of the nodal health agency to undertake the defined task and the empowerment of the inter-sectoral the agency (Planning Commission in this context) to sort out the conflicts. This is an issue waiting to be addressed comprehensively and effectively.

Chapter 4

Government Response

A major initiative has been taken recently by the Government to address a number of issues concerning health governance within the ambit of a single programme. Stung by a barrage of criticism about the non-functioning public health system, the Central government has launched a new programme known as the National Rural Health Mission. In the preamble of the Mission document, major constraints afflicting the public health system have been recognized. These include low level of public health expenditure, lack of community participation in health programmes, inability to integrate sanitation, drinking water and nutrition in the healthcare services, pro-rich subsidization of healthcare expenditure, catastrophic illness leading to indebtedness and poverty of the healthcare seekers, regional inequities in availability of health services, limited synergization of verticalized programmes. The Mission document commits the Government to increase public expenditure on health, provide for a female community health worker for each village, integrate vertical health and family welfare programmes and funds, mainstream ISM & H streams in the public health system, forge effective linkage of the health care services with the social determinants of health, decentralize health programme implementation, bridge intra-state and inter-state disparities in availability of health care facilities and improve access of the people in the rural areas to equitable, affordable, accountable and effective primary healthcare [MoHFW, 2005]. The core strategies crafted for realizing these ambitious objectives include strengthening and upgradation of public health infrastructure, involvement of the Panchayati Raj institutions in health programmes, preparation of the village health plan and inter-sectoral district health plan, technical support to the national, state and district health agencies, formulation of transparent policies for deployment and career development of the health personnel, capacity building for preventive and promotive healthcare, encouragement of the private (non-profit) sector to operate in the under-served areas. The supplementary strategies envisaged for this purpose would strive for regulation of private sector healthcare, promotion of public-private partnership, revitalization of the local health traditions, reorientation of the medical education and provision of social insurance for hospital treatment of the poor.

This framework outlines a strong commitment towards crafting a credible public health system following five key approaches: (a) communitization, (b) adequate and flexible financing, (c) monitoring against IPH standards, (d) innovations in human resource management, (e) building capacity at all levels for decentralized health action (Sinha, 2009). This policy intervention is certainly a welcome initiative. Its importance lies in bringing the crisis-ridden public health system centre stage in the health policy process, taking note of the multi dimensionality of its problems, and incorporating a commitment to address them. The Mission specifically focuses on 18 weak states and the north eastern region. The document has also outlined a plan of action in respect of each objective and set for itself time-bound goals of achieving effective improvements. These goals specifically take into account the Millennium Development Goals (MDGs) settled at the global level. The State governments are required to enter into a MoU (Memorandum of Understanding) with the Central government committing themselves to discharge their role as per the plan of action and its time frame and ensure a minimum of 10% increase in the state budget for public health each year. The State governments, in turn, will receive additional fund, drugs and other material used in the public healthcare from the Centre.

As can be observed, the canvas of the Mission is quite wide, virtually covering major issues of health governance discussed in this paper. The efforts at wide consultation with civil society organizations and advocacy groups in designing the framework and contents of this programme had preceded its launching. Vigorous measures were taken to institutionalize Mission structures and activities more intensively than observed in any programme so far. The intervention is to be appreciated for its attempt to tackle important deficiencies in the primary healthcare in a comprehensive and integrated rather than a piecemeal manner. The pace of implementation at the Central level has also been equally energetic, as can be seen in the pressure exerted on the state governments through intensive monitoring and frequent field inspections by the Central government officials and yearly evaluation by the composite teams of experts and civil society representatives. Separately, experts, social activists and NGOs have been engaged in operationalizing complex social goals of the Mission activities. It would be anxiously watched how the objectives outlined in the Mission statement get translated on the ground in terms of the transformation of the public health system and accrual of the needed benefits to the people.

Notwithstanding the preparatory and operational measures outlined above, serious questions were raised about the framework of the Mission itself when it was launched. A veteran public health expert has critiqued it for not learning from history. Given the complexity of issues plaguing public health system, the approach of the Mission in tackling them is considered simplistic, based as it is on questionable premises (Banerjee, 2005). The existing framework of the health programmes and their structures which have failed to deliver have been left untouched. The proposed approach to effecting architectural correction in the sick public health system continues to remain fragmented rather than integrated (JSA, 2008). The Mission has continued with the World Bank schematic design of creating parallel and vertical management structures for administration of the Mission activities superimposed on the horizontal multiple tiers of governance of the existing health organization. Far from smoothening the governance problems and achieving efficiency in providing necessary and timely inputs to the healthcare facilities, this style of management would add to the problems of achieving coordination and cohesion in a system which is afflicted with distortions created by multiple funding sources with each financing agency devising its own mechanism of allocation of funds, making decisions on programme execution, flow of information, monitoring and reporting (Mittal, 2008). The resultant tensions would detract from the focused attention on improving the delivery of services as per the Mission charter. The Mission also imports the American model of trained managerial physicians to provide leadership in the administration of health services, the relevance of which is doubtful. The approach itself tends to divert attention from the issues of substance to those of management. The Mission's assumption about optimization of resources through this arrangement seems to be misplaced. It would only add to the cost of delivery, problems of coordination and synergisation besides generating tensions within the health organization. The imprint of the donor-driven approach to programme management can be clearly seen in this design even though the Mission is described as 'an entirely home grown idea' developed by the public health experts and external financing for the project has been denied (Sinha, 2009). But the public health system is cluttered with-donor financed programmes and more such projects seem to be in the pipeline (Ashtaker, 2008).

Coming to the delivery of services, the most publicized part of the Mission activities is the provision of a community health worker (ASHA) to act as a bridge between the professionals and the people. This is also the first step towards communitization of the public health delivery system. The community health worker model was implemented in the late 1970s but failed due to the caste/class-based rural power structure (Reddy et al., 2006) and lack of interest, if not hostility of the medical professionals. The community health worker, ASHA, in any case, cannot compensate for the non-functional Sub Centres and ANMs and is not even intended to do so. However, the communitization ethos of ASHA has to be sharply embedded in her role so as not to reduce her to the lowest chain in the hierarchy of service providers. For this worker to carry out its functions meaningfully, what is required is not only a careful process of selection in order that the appointee is acceptable to and easily approachable by diverse social groups in the village community but also a programme of sustained capacity building which prepares her to render healthcare assistance and discharge complex social role. As a health worker, she needs to be empowered with sufficient knowledge of work. The role of a community activist would involve imparting skills for articulating the needs of the community and social mobilization. She also requires to shed social biases, learn from experiences of the people, subject her conduct to their scrutiny and deal with the rural power structure. There is also a need for clarity in the role of ASHA which is distinct from the Anganwadi worker and ANM in order that she is not seen as an adversary of the former and merely an assistant for carrying out the errands of the latter. It should also be both creative as well as within the limits of her capacity to avoid overloading. Out of the eight tasks assigned to ASHA, she is, at present, mainly engaged in the delivery cases and gathering children for immunization which narrows the focus on RCH (Ashtaker, 2008). On the other hand, enlargement of her responsibility to include detection of leprosy cases, etc. is perceived by experts to be beyond her capacity in view of the professional knowledge it requires and also conflicts with her RCH work which involves social activism (George, 2009). Even in terms of the role already defined, the existing capacity building is weak in training, accredition, drug kit refill, not to speak of managing the complex social role. In the absence of a male health activist, her capacity to attend to the health problems of men would be limited (Ashtaker, 2008). Besides, the denial of any financial remuneration to ASHA would militate against the dedication needed for her work and would also be unethical. This cannot be substituted by incentive money for mobilizing pregnant women for institutional delivery, which, in any case, turns out to be very low.

Of the major deficiencies in the existing public health units, human resource management is the most important. Its complex dimensions such as non-availability of service providers, disinclination of the doctors/specialists/paramedics to work in the rural areas, inadequacy of training arrangements, rigid eligibility norms and system of selection for entry into the medical education programmes, mismatch in deployment pattern of the health personnel are deep rooted and require structural change. The Mission has, no doubt, added 2500 specialists, 10,000 doctors, 40,000 ANMS and nurses during the last three years besides using Ayush doctors which has enabled some health centres to provide 24 × 7 services. The compulsory rural postings of medical graduates before post-graduation is another step in this direction (Sinha, 2009). But these measures are not likely to neutralize the dislike for rural jobs due to low salaries, contractual nature of appointments and poor infrastructure and working conditions (Ashtaker, 2008). But the ad hoc measures to address this problem which also include hiring professionals from private sector health establishments, multi-skilling of the existing staff using Ayush doctors as substitutes, are an attempt at fire fighting. They seem to avoid radical reforms in the curricula, mode of training and system of selection for entrants to the medical education which is at the root of it and also fail to address the issue of poaching of professionals from public health centres by the private health sector through strong regulation.

The integration of various health programmes has been effected by bringing them under the umbrella of NRHM in line with the commitment towards their synergistic implementation. Separate societies, each dealing with disease control programmes, have been merged into a single society at the state and district levels. But their operational structures continue to retain their exclusivist and vertical character. No sign of their horizontal merger with the general health set-up is yet in evidence on the ground. This will not happen unless the separate structures of these programmes are dismantled and their workers assigned to the PHCs and CHCs.

The continued excessive focus on reproductive health with its bias for institutional deliveries limits the level of tasks which the institutions of primary healthcare are expected to handle and diverts their attention from numerous health problems which people, including women, face It proceeds on the unsubstantiated assumption that the institutional deliveries per se would reduce MMR (Maternal Mortality Rate). The contribution of institutional deliveries to the reduction in infant and maternal mortality has no solid evidentiary basis and is overrated. The IMR and MMR cannot be reduced unless more fundamental issues of malnutrition and anaemia are comprehensively tackled and effective home-based antenatal and neonatal care is ensured. Besides, most deaths of women take place due to causes other than MMR. The excessive focus on MMR continues to carry the legacy of family planning work in the primary healthcare for which the health policy has been criticized for a long time and tends to narrow down the ambit of RCH work itself. Besides, the strong emphasis on institutional deliveries has resulted in increase in such deliveries, which is considered as the greatest achievement of the NRHM. The institutional delivery itself is driven by financial incentives rather than genuine inclination of the women in labour in the villages to go to the hospitals. In the absence of fully functional PHCs, it has clogged the FRUs (First Referral Units) with simpler cases of delivery to the neglect of more serious cases which they could have attended to. The lure of incentives has also led, at times, to unsafe deliveries since the facilities to reach hospital in time do not exist in most places and there is uncertainty of getting a proper bed. The transport and distance problems in the case of many rural areas are formidable and continue to inhibit the needy women from approaching the healthcare units for treatment. This 'demand side financing' is creating distortions in access to and utilization of healthcare and is not only unsustainable but counter-productive Some critics have also observed that Janani Suraksha Yojana and its emphasis on institutional deliveries is undermining the institution of trained birth attendants and disowning traditional Dais who still handle a substantial number of delivery cases in the rural areas. Though the criticism is officially repudiated as the NRHM does allow for training and skill development of traditional medical attendants wherever they have basic literacy and are willing to do long-term programmes that help them to improve their skills (Sinha, 2009), the conditionality would be difficult to satisfy in many cases. In any case, it would be imprudent for the public health system not to devalue this skilled service provider when effective referral arrangements and emergency services have not yet emerged as alternatives.

The design of NRHM is inadequate in creating a credible and effective arrangement for promoting greater convergence among social development sectors which determine health outcomes like water, sanitation, education and nutrition. The objective is sought to be achieved by constituting a village health and sanitation committee, organizing a village health and nutrition day every month at the ICDS centre and preparation of inter-sectoral district health plan. This creates the impression that the absence of integration is a local problem and an institutional arrangement at a local level would be in a position to forge this convergence. But the fragmentation of social determinants of health is rooted in the structure of the Government at the Central and state levels and centralization and verticalization of the concerned sectoral programmes. Unless this fragmentation is neutralized both institutionally and programmatically at these levels through appropriate interventions, no initiative at the village level or coordination at the district level would yield any meaningful result.

The community participation in health programmes lacks conceptual clarity in terms of a defined framework, contents of what it entails and processes by which it would be promoted. The NRHM is reported to have requested the most 'independent minded non-governmental organizations (NGOs)' to create a framework for community monitoring by organizing public hearings and to make public health system accountable (Sinha, 2009). At present, communitization has been effected under the umbrella of the PRIs by constituting village health and Sanitation Committees and facility specific Rogi Kalyan Samitis (RKSs) for PHCs, CHCs, Sub-district and District hospitals. But there is little by way of community involvement in the management of healthcare services in the deliberations of the VHSCs except operation of joint bank account and organizing a Health and Nutrition Day. The NRHM has also permitted other village-level organizations such as SHGs Water users association, Mahila Samakhya to be represented in the VHSCs while the civil society has been given representation in the RKSs. How this cluttering of diverse functional groups would promote communitisation remains to be seen. But it seems problematic conceptually and structurally. As for the Rogi Kalyan Samitis, this institutional arrangement continues to be perceived and function as an alternative financing arrangement with emphasis on collection of user charges rather than an instrument of facilitating access of the poorer sections and exercising social control over the healthcare delivery (NRHM, 2007). They are far removed from being an instrument upholding the interests of the community, which obviously implies the disempowered larger mass of people. The community participation in its wider sense, implies social control over the entire domain of health activities at the local level. Viewed thus, it is a potentially radical measure which can change the entire structure and processes of health planning and delivery of services. In the unfolding of Mission activities, it gets bureaucratically designed and implemented. It has been reduced to an arrangement where the health professionals give lectures to the members of the committee or the PRIs or even arrange occasional public hearing. No genuine and assertive community involvement is likely to emerge from such a conception of its role and structure. It is hoped that a proper framework of communitization would come up from the NGOs entrusted with this task

Connected with the issue of community participation is the phenomenon of social exclusion which the marginalized sections of the society face. The design of NRHM has no focus on the socially marginalized sections which suffer a variety of exclusionary experiences in accessing health services. The social barriers of caste, ethnicity, religion, gender and disability continue to inhibit the sections of society from getting the desired benefits of health services. This is evident from the documentary evidence that is available as well as the health profile of these groups. The Mission has not adopted specific strategies to counteract these barriers by way of programme content, attitudinal orientation of medical staff, and other creative instruments to improve their access to health services and enhance their utilization for promoting good health.

The critique of NRHM has also contested the element of 'flexibility' in its operations considering that the design and budgeting of programmes leaves little creative freedom for the states to develop requisite political will and strategies for tackling health problems of their people. There is also a mismatch between local needs and NRHM prescriptions. The Mission has also been faulted for tardy and ineffective utilization of funds as also the financing model of flow of funds to the States and then to district societies. The latter makes financial expenditure unaccountable since it bypasses the prescribed procedures of scrutiny (Ashtaker, 2008). The Mission has, however, rebutted this view as flexibility has been provided to the States to design their own interventions for outreach of services. Several states have adopted innovative locally relevant strategies which indicate a diversity of interventions. The untied funds made available to committees at different levels have enabled them to spend the money under community supervision on items as per local need which have improved public health services (Sinha, 2009). The irony is that many committees are hesitant to use this flexibility of decentralized spending for fear of scrutiny which underlines the need for necessary training and confidence building. The Mission has also dispelled the impression that transfer of funds to societies bypassing the treasury system makes expenditure unaccountable as the societies are also subject to the normal audit as also the audit of Comptroller and Auditor General. The arrangement of flow of funds to societies directly was necessitated due to the delays caused in transfer of funds from states to implementing agencies through the treasury system (Sinha, 2009).

The Mission has completed less than three years, which is a short time to evaluate its impact. In terms of the limited focus on incremental improvements, progress has been registered in out-patient cases, institutional deliveries, immunization, drug availability, diagnostic and ambulance services, etc. (Sinha, 2009). The First Common Review Mission carried out in November 2007 also candidly brought out a number of deficiencies. These included continued staffing gaps, little inclination in the state governments to abolish private practice of doctors in the public health system, shortage of essential drugs and irregular supplies, lack of transport and infrastructure, unsatisfactory maintenance, sub-optimal utilization of the facilities, inadequate training and skill development of the existing staff, distortions in the selection process, inadequacy in capacity building and lack of clear articulation of responsibilities in respect of the ASHAs, poor internalization of IPH standards in terms of output to be delivered, slow pace of integration between different divisions of health department, weak community participation both in planning and delivery of health services, inadequate progress in decentralization and absence of any measures for bio-waste management. The CRM conceded that the peripheral healthcare institutions—Sub Centers, PHCs—do not show any visible improvement (NRHM, 2007). Perhaps the second CRM which was carried out at the end of last year may have achieved greater progress and, in the coming years, the Mission may fare still better. But the larger question is whether the Mission has the potential of transforming the public health system without pursuing structural changes to correct the cumulative adverse effect of past interventions? Also, whether even incremental improvements registered during the life of the Mission can be sustained in the absence of strong political pressure from the large sections of people who are deprived of the elementary health services. The perspective presented in this paper makes it difficult to sustain optimism on either. As for the former, the Mission does not even make this bold claim. Major governance problems will continue to persist.

Chapter 5

Dynamics of Health Sector Governance

The health sector is overburdened with governance issues which have severely affected the design of health planning and delivery of health services. Health sector governance has been problematic since Independence and can be related to various pressures exerted on the state which influenced its decision making. These pressures emanated from the political and bureaucratic elites, medical professionals, external agencies and commercial interests. The pressures from political/bureaucratic elites have been largely directed towards cornering resources for establishing, expanding and improving health facilities in the urban areas, developed rural pockets and constituencies of the people with high political clout. This was responsible for the neglect of underserved, remote and inaccessible areas and underdeveloped regions and efforts to improve the health of poor and socially marginalized sections. The political elite interferes with the rational location of the healthcare units, norm-based deployment of medical personnel and efficient procurement of drugs and consumables, etc. to serve its narrow political interests. The influence of medical professionals aided by commercialization of medicine has created a monopoly of the Western over other systems of medicine. This unequal distribution of power within the system of medicine enables the allopathic stream of professionals to assert their superiority, debunk other streams of medicine as unscientific, and appropriate most of the public resources, development opportunities and decision-making positions. Their clout emboldens them to dictate terms of their own engagement. They refuse rural postings, resist abolition of private practice, oppose restructuring of the medical education curricula suited to the needs of the people, ridicule measures to use low-cost technology and least-cost medicine, and promote expansion of hospital-based medicine and hi-tech specialization. These medical professionals sabotage decentralization of healthcare, deride appropriate integration of different medicine systems, frustrate efforts to transfer knowledge to the community health workers and show little interest in the widespread dissemination of health education to the people.

The commercial interests have thwarted attempts to regulate the drug industry in terms of production structure, distributional arrangements, margin of profit and pricing norms and check the practice of irrational, unsafe and expensive medicine. These interests have been instrumental in getting the pharmaceutical industry de-regulated and protection available to the public sector production units removed. The private health sector has extracted concessions—fiscal, infrastructural, financial for its growth but has refused to abide by the contractual obligation to provide free healthcare to the specified percentage of poor patients in return. It has also lobbied to get liberalized policy instruments in its favour to tap the growth opportunities and maximize profits in the new economic order.

The pressure from external agencies can be observed in the centralized and verticalized health programmes [Malaria and Small Pox in the pre-reforms period], character of medical education and framing of its curricula on the lines followed in the developed countries, push given to a barrage of global programmes initiated through the international organizations, assignment of an overriding priority to the family planning programme in health planning and pattern of production, distribution, prescription and pricing of drugs. These pressures have persuaded the Government to implement a frenzied, prolonged and exhausting pulse polio drive under the cover of polio eradication. The external commercial interests have also intensively lobbied to get new and exorbitantly expensive vaccines—Hepatitis B (Dasgupta, 2006) and Pneumococcal vaccine included in the basket of immunization which is not justified by any objective evaluation of priority, equity and affordability when even the existing six vaccines in EPI

(Extended Programme of Immunization) reach only 50% of the population (Puliyel, 2008). Their impact has been most marked in the production of health manpower unsuited to the local needs, reduced autonomy in the health policy process, pattern of drug production unaffordable to the people and the prioritization of health programmes unrelated to the objective norms and design of their management which prevents horizontal integration at the local level and causes dysfunctionalities in the health organization. The cumulative effects of these pressures have posed multiple challenges to governance in the health sector.

Since economic reforms began from the mid-1980s, India has committed itself to progressively integrate with the global economy as a part of its paradigm shift towards neo-liberalism in macro-economic management. This requires India to open up its economy to national and international capital and focus on the primacy of economic growth. The private sector is the pivot of this growth vehicle which demands enabling conditions to achieve this objective. With encouragement from promotional policies pursued by the Government, the private sector healthcare has already emerged as the dominant supplier of curative healthcare. The integration with global economy has made it one of the fastest growing sectors in the country. The Government is, therefore, obliged to let this sector achieve its optimum growth potential through various policy instruments. With this strategic position, the private sector is influencing design of the health policy and the process of governance. The private sector growth in the healthcare segment is instrumental in creating iniquitous healthcare arrangements—different standards of health services catering to service seekers with differential purchasing capacity. The profit orientation of private healthcare also gives rise to unethical and irrational practices and exploitative nature of treatment. The sound governance of the health sector would demand that this sector be regulated to promote equity. This would, however, make the governance problematic because it is difficult to strike a balance between the demand for facilitating private sector growth and the imperative of curbing its operations and accumulative instincts to provide justice to the people. The difficulty gets compounded as the autonomy of state in devising policy instruments for rendering justice to the people is severely circumscribed by the clout of private sector in the country as well as the pressure of global capital and institutions. Its action, therefore, cannot go against their interests.

This indication is already available from the measures proposed to promote equity against the increasing cost of healthcare. To make health facilities affordable to the people, health insurance is being promoted. Besides those who can contribute towards their own insurance, social health insurance has been envisaged for the workers in the unorganized sector and the people below poverty line. A National Health Insurance Scheme called the Rashtriya Swasthya Bima Yojna has recently been announced which provides Rs.30,000 'in patient' benefit at a premium of Rs. 600, which the Government pays if the person is poor (Das, 2008). The recently enacted Un-organized Workers Social Security Act, 2008 has also incorporated this scheme in its ambit. This solution targets not the reduction in cost of treatment but the mode of its financing. The solution is welcome to the private sector as it increases its business without hurting profitability. But the provision for meeting hospitalization cost through insurance would fail to ensure that healthcare is easily accessible and affordable to the poorer sections due to a variety of constraints. At the same time, it would create newer governance problems arising from the interface of the poor with the service providing organizations and insurance companies. In short, the neo-liberal policy frame compels the state to use the very instrument of the market to solve the problem of inequity which itself is rooted in the operation of market forces.

The health governance in the global economy paradigm is getting enmeshed in the ever-increasing contradictions of policies pursued in different sectors. A classic example is the conflict between trade and health policy. The situation of non-availability of doctors in the rural areas requires the state to regulate its migration policy for medical and para-medical professionals and to change the medical education and training to conform to the needs of rural areas. But the trade policy in the 'services' sector of the economy compels it to vigorously promote export of health manpower and to reorient medical syllabi to suit the international market. The corporatization of healthcare and promotion of medical tourism encourage brain drain and brain skimming from the public health units which adversely affects their services. The state has to allow free flow of health-threatening products, e.g. junk food, cola drinks and even their aggressive advertisement under the compulsion of free trade regime even though their consumption creates an enormous burden on its healthcare services. The genetically modified products whose consequences on the health of people are unpredictable in the short run are also being permitted to be marketed in the country on the same grounds. In the latter case, the Supreme Court has intervened on a PIL to monitor the field trials of genetically modified seeds of some crops where the Government has resolutely supported the interests of the multi-national seed companies. A similar conflict has been thrown up between the health policy and the pharmaceutical policy to which a reference has been made earlier. There are numerous areas of such conflict.

The global policy making has also undermined the state's capacity to govern the health sector because its sovereignty is compromised and autonomy considerably reduced. Its public health policy is driven by multilateral and bilateral agencies and associated academic institutions and corporate interests by directing international resources (Murugaswamipillay, 1994). It has lost its maneuverability to intervene in the health sector in the same manner as it used to do in the pre-reforms period. It is required to accommodate health policy changes pushed in by the global organizations (World Bank, UNICEF, WHO, WTO) within its national policy profile since they are backed by powerful global interests. It has no option to get out of such commitments even if their pursuit turns out to have adverse implications for the people. The global programmes and their prioritization is one such part of the policy. The programme for eradication of polio through campaign mode as a high priority concern, for example, was imposed by these global interests. It could not have been justified in terms of our epidemiological priorities, socio-economic conditions and available infrastructure and resources. This programme has claimed disproportionate financial and manpower resources, pushed back immunization for five vaccine preventable diseases, and has adversely affected the implementation of other health programmes. It is now being realized that it would be difficult to eradicate polio given our socio-economic conditions despite the repeated doses administered to the target groups which throw up sporadic polio cases. But the drive continues nonetheless. The adverse health effects of repeated doses of oral polio vaccine are getting exposed but are deliberately ignored by the Government and the media. The continuation of pulse polio programme cannot be justified as our national priority. But the state does not have the courage to opt out of it. It is, in fact, suppressing information about the cases adversely affected by repeated polio drops (Sathyamala et al., 2006; Mittal et al., 2006).

The de-politicization of health governance arising out of the imperative of globalization has enormously increased the power of the national elites and delegitimized democratic institutions. The global public-private partnerships have emerged as parallel health governance institutions. They design and prioritize health programmes which are required to be implemented by the nations (Mittal, 2005). These programmes tend to draw resources—financial and manpower—from other programmes by displacing local priorities. Similarly, the rulings of WTO may involve the risk of removing/changing legal provisions, policies and practices already in operation if they are perceived to come in the way of free flow of trade. The member nations of WTO have to comply with its directions for fear of sanctions imposed on them (Bertrand et al., 2001; Retallack, 2001). This pattern of health policy making has no element of political participation and does not respond to the local needs. It is designed by the international technocrats and other interests and reinforced by the global governance institutions—WB, WHO, WTO, etc. who have no accountability for the adverse health outcomes these policies and programmes may generate (Buse et al., 2002). The national and local political institutions and processes are irrelevant to the dynamics of globalized policy making. These structures and processes are merely used for getting policy endorsement post facto. This has resulted in the de-legitimization of democratic processes and the alienation of democratic institutions from the people. In such a situation, the national elites, (bureaucratic, technocratic, commercial) become very powerful as they align with the global forces and present the policy crafted in global arena as 'inevitable' from which the country cannot back off. The complexity of the global economy and its processes have also made the average political leader ill-equipped to contest their presentation. This deprives the health governance of the acutely needed political direction for ensuring access of the people to health services, equity, the healthcare arrangements and quality of care rendered therein for achieving improved health outcomes for them.

Chapter 6

Health Governance: The Two Paradigms

That the health sector faces serious governance problems is not in doubt. These problems have arisen due to a number of factors unique to our situation. First, the health policy that emerged after Independence was not shaped by the demands or visions of a political movement nor it was the culmination of a struggle involving conflict of class interests. Unlike England, for example, where the pressures exerted by worker's unions led to the introduction of the National Health Service (Navarro, 1978), the healthcare arrangements in independent India were established by a decision emanating from the report of an expert body, the Bhore Committee, endorsed by the interim Government shortly before the end of colonial rule. It reflected the aspirations of national leaders and, in the absence of any opposition to it, may be perceived to have reflected the national consensus. Health governance also cannot be entirely de-linked from its colonial past. The internal organization of medicine, the system of health facilities, the nature and content of medical education, etc. continue to be rooted in the colonial practices. The provision of health services has also to contend with institutions, structures and processes of society marked by sharp inequalities of economic class, social status and political power. The paradigm of global economy and nature of development defined by it too had a great deal of impact on the design of health policy and range of services flowing from it. The external intervention in the health sector, though insubstantial, also influenced health governance through the leverage of financial and technical assistance. While politics and its processes contributed to the style of governance in the health sector during this phase, the strength of commercial interests set the limits to its potential reach and effectiveness. Is there any overarching conceptual framework which links these explanations to situate the roots of health governance problems?

The health policy and governance in a modern state is usually explained in terms of the 'power-elite paradigm' according to which major happenings in the organization of medicine result from the manipulations of specific interest groups. The medical professionals occupy the dominant position in these groups. The manipulations are directly related to the interests served by interventions in the system of medicine. "The professionals who provide health (medical) services have critical roles in the health system… (given the nature of modern medicine) they will continue to influence if not, indeed, dominate the health sector... health provider sits at the centre of the system... and this centrality of the function is a source of power over all other actors' (Bjorkman, 1991). The power of medical professionals is related to their organizational strength and capacity to use their expertise in the policies of decision making on health. The medical professionals are 'well organized... exercise large professional and political powers and their professional interests are firmly established in the legal, political and financial systems... any attempt to reform the medical sector at large will have to reckon with their institutional dominance' [Bovens et al., 2001]. This is because the medical professionals are the major beneficiaries of resources in the health sector as well as key decision makers in their allocation.

This paradigm is challenged by an alterative paradigm which positions medical professionals in the dominant class in society at the centre of political power. The actions of medical professionals are aligned with the interests of this class which is locked in conflict with other classes in society. This class struggle provides the basis for growth and distribution of health services. In a capitalist or mixed economy, the health policy and governance would reflect the arrangement arrived at between the social demands on health services made by different sections of the poor and social needs of the dominant class to accommodate them since the primary struggle is between these two classes. The professional interests do not shape or influence that compromise. The state merely gives effect to it. Its actions are tilted in favour of the interests of the dominant class (Navarro, 1978).

We shall examine if the governance issues in the health sector in India are illuminated by these seemingly conflicting paradigms or whether a third paradigm can provide a more convincing explanation of the problems encountered. Roger Jeffrey seems to have articulated the 'power-elite' paradigm in his book *The Politics of Health in India* (Jeffrey, 1988). In his view, the medical professionals have become central to the health policy and governance. They have used their expertise as a political weapon to influence the decisions taken on health services from time to time. Along with the colonial legacy of supremacy conferred on Western medicine, the nature of politics in independent India also helped in enhancing the position of medical professional. The absence of a strong working class and deficiency of organizations representing the poor prevented raising of health problems on ideological lines projecting their interests. This enabled the ruling elite to speak on their behalf. The political processes in the circumstances created the space for professionals to place themselves strategically and to manipulate decision making to their advantage. No coherent alternative paradigm contesting this explanation has come up in the public discourse or academic literature in the country. The design of health policy after Independence was usually viewed as a product of the enlightened orientation of political elite and the influence of socialist thought on the post-colonial governance in the country. However, in the early decades of independence, the overall governability of the state (not in the context of the health sector) was under considerable scrutiny and widely commented upon by the Western academics. The governance problems encountered by the post-colonial state in India were attributed to its inherent incapacity to take hard decisions, its vulnerability to the pressures of organized interests and its ineffectiveness in implementing laws and policies which were characteristics of a 'soft state' (Myrdal, 1970). Varying versions of this characterization were articulated by others (Kohli, 1990; Rudolf and Rudolf, 1987). This explanation virtually provided substance to the power elite paradigm as the elite power circumscribed the state's capacity to govern effectively, thereby turning it into a soft apparatus.

The discourse on health problems in this paper would indicate that the 'power elite' paradigm does not illuminate governance problems in the health sector. In the current situation, it is more than evident that the interests of 'capital' represented by industrial and business elite are central to the health policy and its implementation. The capital is the prime mover of growth not only of the economy but also its health segment. This can be observed in the pace of its growth which is faster than any other sector. The interests of 'capital' have an edge over public interest in as much as their concerns cannot be disregarded by the Government. The interests of professional groups, bureaucratic and political elite, coincide with the interests of capital and, therefore, are quite sub-served by latter's hegemonic position. Both support the current paradigm of health development planning pushed by the existing global order and effectively steered by the global governance institutions—World Bank, IMF, WHO, UNICEF, WTO. There is no discordance in their approach. Rather, there is a convergence of interests of groups involved in promoting private sector led healthcare. The professional elite favours it as it enhances opportunities for generating higher income and expanding career development opportunities. The bureaucratic and political elite gains in terms of sophisticated healthcare on a par with the one available in the developed countries. The capital through its enormous power forges this consensus for its own penetration and expansion. Its primary interest is to marginalize, if not altogether destroy, public healthcare (curative) so as to occupy that space. The state is just an instrument of implementing this consensus since taken together, this combine of interests constitutes the class which wields overwhelming power. The resistance only comes from the poor (working class and other categories of socially and economically marginalized sections). But they are too weak to pose any threat to the combined strength of above forces backed by the state. This, in our view, is the 'paradigm' which Vicente Navarro articulated with reference to the NHS of the UK.

How does this explain, one may ask, the pre-reforms governance, since the private sector in healthcare was not a dominant player then? The answer lies in the shifting interests of the national and international capital in the two phases: In the pre-reforms phase, the 'capital' was interested in public investment for expansion of healthcare facilities to create necessary infrastructure, demand for healthcare, production of trained manpower and enunciation of promotive fiscal policies which it could later use for its growth. It was not interested in making this investment because it would not have earned necessary profit in that phase both for lack of demand and low purchasing power of the people. It needed public health services for the working class and the very poor in order that it could absolve itself of the responsibility for providing 'affordable' healthcare to them and a minimum level of satisfaction of healthcare needs for its workers to pursue unhindered expansion. The role of professionals was to promote a model of healthcare which would open up opportunities for its own expansion, career development and consolidation of power in the system for which investment in healthcare was needed. The state alone was in a position to do so at that stage. The bureaucratic and political power elite also supported the state-funded healthcare because the people needed it and private sector showed no interest in providing it. Also, it was easier to corner this investment for setting up infrastructure in areas of their influence and to grab educational and job opportunities for their relations. A working class with a minimum level of subsistence was necessary to lay the foundation for capital-led economic growth for production of drugs, equipments and consumables. The state-funded healthcare was a part of this subsistence package. Thus, the interests of capital, professionals, bureaucratic and political elites converged. The poorer sections did not present any opposition to it because, after the total neglect during the colonial period, they were assured of some healthcare free of cost. But all this changed because of the ascendancy of neo-liberalism world wide, growth of the private sector, Structural Adjustment Programme, health sector reforms and the globalization of

Indian economy. As the impact of these changes began to be experienced, the conflict between the interests of poor and those of capital started growing. This has crystallized the 'class struggle' in the area of health policy and governance as evident from the issues thrown up.

The Nature of state

What is the character of 'state' that emerges through the lens of this governance dynamics? The post-colonial development state in India with its 'welfare-centric' economy was viewed as 'soft' as it lacked the toughness and effectiveness necessary for governability. Has this pattern of governance changed with the neo-liberal transformation of economy and, if so, in what direction? Irrespective of whether one concurs in labelling the state as 'soft' in the pre-reforms phase, the state, notwithstanding its vulnerability to pressures from various segments of the dominant social class, was relatively more alive to the social demands of the poor (though ineffective in accommodating them). The 'post-reforms' state has distinctly become unresponsive to the needs and interests of this class and closed to the scrutiny and review of its health policy paradigm despite the mounting evidence of adverse health outcomes for them on this account. (The NRHM intervention does not reverse this policy). It is easily 'amenable' to pressures of the dominant social class in collaboration with the external actors backed by global economic forces more than ever before. But it feels less obligated to accommodate the interests of the working class and poorer sections (not taking into account the minor sops thrown at them under the pressure of electoral compulsion). It perceives little threat from them due to their weak position in the absence of strong political forces to mobilize them on health issues. Thus, it has acquired a Janus-faced character, servile to the dominant social class but tough in resisting any challenge from and on behalf of the poor to the conceptual framework of its policy and operations flowing from it. But this is precisely what makes the situation propitiate for a sharper conflict to emerge between the contending classes. The health sector, therefore, would now emerge, more clearly, as an arena of intense ideological struggle which would facilitate political mobilization of the poor and working class along their 'vision' of health and its determinants for counteracting the widening inequities in access to healthcare and other health benefits. The outcome of this struggle would shape a more equitable and humane health policy and provide the needed political direction to its governance.

References

Ashtaker, Shyam, 'The National Rural Health Mission: A Stock Taking', *Economic and Political Weekly*, 13 September, 2008.

Bajaj, J.S., *'Medical Education and Health Care'*. Indian Institute of Advanced Study, Simla, 1998.

Banerjee, D., 'Political Economy of Public Health in India', in M. Das Gupta, Lincoln C. Chen and T.N. Krishnan, *Health, Poverty and Development of India*. Oxford, Bombay, 1996.

Banerjee, D., 'Fundamental Shift in the Approach to International Health', by WHO, UNICEF and the World Bank: Instances of the Practice of "Intellectual Fascism" and "Totalitarianism" in some Asian Countries, *International Journal of Health Services*. Vol. 29 (No. 2), 1999.

Banerjee, D., 'Politics of Rural Health in India', *Economic and Political Weekly*, 23 July, 2005.

Baru, Rama, 'Mixed Economy in Health Care: Some Issues', *IASSI Quarterly*, July, 1995.

Baru, Rama, *'Private Health Care in India: Social Characteristics and Trends'*. Sage, New Delhi, 1990.

Baru, Rama and Amar Jessani, 'The Role of the World Bank in International Health: Renewed Commitment and Partnership', *Social Sciences and Medicine*, Vol. 50, 2000.

Baru, Rama, V., 'Health Sector Reforms and Structural Adjustment: State Level Analysis', in I. Qadeer, K. Sen and K.R. Nayyar (eds.), *Public Health and the Poverty of Reforms*. Sage, New Delhi, 2001.

Bertrand, Agnes and Laurence Kalafitades, 'World Trade Organization and the Liberalization', in Edward Goldsmith and Jerry Mander, *The Case Against the Global Economy and Turn Towards Localization*, Earthscan, London, 2001.

Bhargava, Anurag and S. Srinivasan, 'Availability and Access to Drugs,' in Sujata Prasad and C. Sathyamala (eds.), *Securing Health for All; Dimensions and Challenges*. Institute of Human Development, New Delhi, 2006.

Bhatt, Ramesh, 'The Private/Public Mix in Health Care in India', *Health Policy and Planning*, Vol. 8 (1), 1993.

Bhatt, Ramesh,'Regulation of the Private Health Sector in India', *International Journal of Health Planning and Management*, Vol. 11, 1996.

Bhatt, Ramesh,'A Note on Policy Initiative to Protect the Poor from High Medical Cost', Working Paper, IIM Ahmedabad, November, 1999.

Bhatt, Ramesh, 'Issues in Health: Public-Private Partnership', *Economic and Political Weekly*, 30 December, 2000.

Bjorkman, W.J., 'Conclusion: Grains among the Chaff-rhetoric and Reality' in Alten Settler and Stuart C. Haywood, *Comparative Health Policy and the New Right: From Rhetoric to Reality*, St. Martin Press, NewYork, 1991.

Bose, Ashish and P.B. Desai, *'Studies in Social Dynamics of Primary Health Care'*. Hindustan Publishing Corporation (India), Delhi, 1983.

Bose, A.,'Curbing Female Foeticide: Doctors, Governments and Civil Society Ensure Failure', *Economic and Political Weekly*, 23 February, 2002.

Bovens, Mark, Hart Paul't and Guy B. Peters (eds.), *'Success and Failure in Public Governance – A Comparative Analysis'*. Edward Elgar Publishing, Cheltennam, UK, 2001.

Brass, Paul R., 'India, Myron Weiner and Political Science of Development', *Economic and Political Weekly*, July, 2002.

Buse, Kent, Fustukian Suzanne, Nick Drager and Kelly Lee, *'Globalisation and Health Policy: Trends and Opportunities'*, in Lee Kelly, Fustukian Suzanne and Kent Buse (eds.), *Health Policy in a Globalising World*. Cambridge University Press, 2005.

Chaterjee, Meera, *'Implementing Health Policy'*. Manohar Publications, New Delhi, 1988.

Das, Gurcharan, 'Finally, A Lifeline for India's Poor', *The Times of India*, 2 November, 2008.

Das Jishnu and Jeffrey Hommer, 'Strained Mercy: Quality of Medicare in Delhi', *Economic and Political Weekly*, 28 February, 2004.

Dasgupta, Monica, 'Public Health in India: Dangerous Neglect', *Economic and Political Weekly*, December, 2003.

Dasgupta, Rajib, 'Hepatitis B Vaccination Strategies in India: Questionable Evidence and Powerful Market Forces', in Sujata Prasad and C. Sathyamala (eds.), 2006

Devarayan, Shantayanan and Shekhar Shah, 'Making Services Work for India's Poor', *Economic and Political Weekly*, 28, February, 2004.

Dilip, T.R., 'Extent of Equity in Access to Health Care Services in India' in Gangolli, et al (eds.), 2005.

Duggal, Ravi, 'Public Health Expenditures, Investment and Financing under the Shadow of a Growing Private Sector', in Leena Gangolli, et al (eds.), 2005.

Gangolli, Leena V., Ravi Duggal and Abhay Shukla, *'Review of Health Care in India'*, CEHAT, Mumbai, 2005.

Garg, Charu, 'Is Health Insurance Feasible in India: Issues in Private and Social Health Insurance', in Sujata Prasad and C. Sathyamala (eds.), 2006.

Gautham, Meenakshi, 'Merit versus Social Responsibility', *The Hindu*, July, 2006.

Gill, S.S. and R.H. Ghuman, 'Rural Health: Proactive Role for the State', *Economic and Political Weekly*, 16 December, 2000.

Green, Andrew, 'The State of Health Planning in the 90s', *Health Policy and Planning*, Vol. 10 (i), 1995.

Griffiths, A., 'Economies and Health: Developed Countries', in A. Griffiths and Z. Bankowski (eds.), *Economics and Health Policy*, Council for International Organisation of Medical Sciences and Sondoz Institute for Health and Socio-economic Studies, WHO Publication Centre, Geneva, Albany, New York, 1980.

The Hindu, 'Include Mental Health Issues in Election Manifestoes', 26 March, 2009.

ICSSR–ICMR, 'Health for All: An Alternative Strategy', Indian Institute of Education and ICSSR, Pune, 1981.

Iyer, Aditi and Amar Jessani, *'Medical Ethics'*. Voluntary Health Association of India, New Delhi, 2000.

Jan Swasthya Abhiyan, 'Report of People's Rural Health Watch'. 2008.

Jan Swasthya Abhiyan, 'People's Health Manifesto, 2009: Health for All Now, a call to all political parties', 2009.

Jeffrey, Roger, *'The Politics of Health in India'*. University of California Press, Berkeley, 1988.

Jessani, Amar and Saraswathi Anantharaman, *'Private Sector and Privatisation in the Health Care Services'*. The Foundation for Research in Community Health, Mumbai, 1993.

Kethineni, V., 'Political Economy of State Intervention in Health Care', *Economic and Political Weekly*, 19 October, 199[illegible].

Kohli, Atul, *'Democracy and Discontent: India's Growing Crisis of Governability'*. Cambridge University Press, 1990.

Lavis, John and Terry, Sullivan, 'Governing Health', in D. Drache and T. Sullivan (eds.), *Health Reforms – Public Success and Private Failure*. Routledge, 1999.

Locost, 'Impoverishing the Poor: Pharmaceutical and Drug Pricing in India', Locost, Baroda, 2004.

Ludden, David, 'Developing Regimes in South Asia: History and Governance Conundrum', *Economic and Political Weekly*, 10 September, 2005.

Madan, T.N., *'Doctors and Society: Three Asian Case Studies'*. Vikas Publishing House, New Delhi, 1980.

Mathew, George, 'Lessons for Integration of Health Programmes', *Economic and Political Weekly*, 4 April, 2009.

Mavalankar, Dilip V., 'A Review of Human Resource Management in Relation to RCH Programme in India: Issues and Challenges', IIM, Ahmedabad, Working Paper, 99-01-02, January, 1999.

Menon, Parvathy, 'Kidneys Still for Sale', *Frontline*, 2 February, 2002.

Ministry of Chemicals, Pharmaceutical Policy, 2002.

Ministry of Health and Family Welfare, National Health Policy, 1983.

Ministry of Health and Family Welfare, National Health Policy, 2000[a]

Ministry of Health and Family Welfare, National Policy on Indian Systems of Medicine and Homeopathy, 2002[b].

Ministry of Health and Family Welfare, National Rural Health Mission (2005-2012): Mission Document, 2005.

Mishra, Rajiv, Rachel Chatterjee and Sujatha Rao, *'India Health Report'*. Oxford, New Delhi, 2003.

Mittal, Onkar and C. Sathyamala, 'Global Polio Eradication Initiative in India 1995-2006', Background Information Note for IMA Conference, 4 May, 2006.

Mittal, Onkar, 'International Health Governance in the Era of Imperialist Globalisation', *Revolutionary Democracy*, Vol. XI, No. 1, April, 2005.

Mittal, Onkar, National Rural Health Mission (NRHM): A Critique, paper presented in a seminar on Right Based Entitlements held in Council for Social Development, New Delhi, 2 November, 2008.

Mohanty, Manoranjan, 'Retreat to Governance Under Globalization: Lessons from the Poverty Eradication Experience in Orrissa' in Kameshar Choudhery (ed.), *Globalization, Governance Reforms and Development in India*. Sage, New Delhi, 2007.

Murlidharan, V.R., 'When is Access to Health Care Equal', *Economic and Political Weekly*, 19 June, 1993.

Murlidharan, V.R., 'Technology and Costs of Medical Care: Some Emerging Issues and Policy Imperatives', in Barbara Harris White, and S. Subramanian, (eds.) *Ill fare in India: Essays in India's Social Sector*. Sage, New Delhi, 2001.

Murugaswamipillay, Sivakumar, 'Who Determines Health Policy' in

Felicity T. Cutts and Peter G. Smith (eds.), *Vaccination and World Health*, John Wiley & Sons, Chichester, U.K., 1994.

Myrdal, Gunnar, *'Challenge of World Poverty'*. Vintage, Middlesex, U.K., 1971.

Nandraj, Sunil, 'Beyond the Law and the Lord: Quality of Private Health Care', *Economic and Political Weekly*, 2 July, 1994.

Nandraj, S. and Ravi Duggal, *'Financing of Disease Control Programmes'*, CEHAT, Mumbai, 1996.

Nandraj, S. and Ravi Duggal, *'Physical Standards in the Private Health Sector'*, CEHAT, Mumbai, 1996.

National Rural Health Mission, The Common Review Mission, 2007.

Navarro, Vicente, *'Class Struggle, the State and Medicine'*. Watson Publication International, New York, 1978.

Oomen, T.K., 'Health Policy and Medical Education in India', in S.K. Lal and Ambika Chandani (eds.), *Medical Care: Readings in Medical Sociology*. University of Rajasthan, Jaipur, 1987.

Palaniswamy, K.R., 'Rescue Modern Medicine from its Traps', *The Hindu*, 15 June, 2006.

Patnaik, Ila, 'India's Ailing Public Health Service', *Financial Express*, 4 July, 2006.

Planning Commission, The Tenth Five Year Plan, 2002.

Prasad, Sujata and C. Sathyamala (eds.), *'Securing Health For All; Dimensions and Challenges'*, Institute of Human Development, New Delhi, 2006.

Priya, R., 'Disability Adjusted Life Years as a Tool for Public Health Policy: A Critical Assessment' in I. Qadeer, K. Sen and K.R. Nayyar, (eds.), *Public Health and the Poverty of Reforms*. Sage, New Delhi, 2001[a].

Priya, Ritu, 'Towards Health Security for Women and Children: Exploring Debates and Options', in Sujata Prasad and C. Sathyamala (eds.), 2001[b].

Public Health Resource Network, 'Introduction to Public Health System', State Health Resource Centre, Chhatisgarh, 2006.

Puliyel, Jacob, 'Seeking Problems for Solutions', A Paper presented in the Seminar on Right Based Entitlement, held in Council for Social Development on 6-7 November, 2008.

Qadeer, Imrana, 'Health Services System in India: An Expression of Socio-Economic Inequalities', *Social Action*, Vol. 3-5, July-September, 1985.

Qadeer, Imrana, 'Primary Health Care: A Paradise Lost', *IASSI Quarterly*, Vol. 14, Nos. 1 & 2, 1995.

Qadeer, Imrana, 'Health Care Systems in Transition III', *Journal of Public Health Medicine*, Vol. 22, No. 1, 2000.

Qadeer, Imrana, K. Sen and K.R. Nayyar (eds.), *'Public Health and Poverty of Reforms'*. Sage, New Dehi, 2001.

Qadeer, Imrana, 'Debt Payment and Devaluing Elements of Public Health', *Economic and Political Weekly*, 19 November, 2002.

Raghuram, N., 'N. Raghuram and others Vs Union of India and others', a PIL filed in the Supreme Court in December, 2008 challenging this order.

Reddy, M. Gopinath, K. Jayalakshmi and Anne-Marie Goetz, 'Politics of Pro-poor Reform in Health Sector', *Economic and Political Weekly*, 4 February, 2006.

Retallack, Simon, 'The Environmental Cost of Economic Globalisation', in E. Goldsmith and J. Mander (eds.), *The Case Against the Global Economy and for a Turn Towards Localization*. Earthscan, London, 2001.

Rifkin, Susan B., *'Health Planning and Community Participation: Case Studies in South-East Asia'*. Croom Helm, London, 1985.

Rudolph, L.I. and S.H. Rudolph, *'In Pursuit of Lakshmi: Political Economy of the Indian State'*. Orient Longman, New Delhi, 1987.

Sagar, Alpna, 'Reproduction Health Package: A Chimera for Women's Health', in Imrana Qadeer, et al (eds.), 2001.

Sathyamala, C. and Onkar Mittal, 'Polio Eradication Initiative at What Cost?', in Sujata Prasad and C. Sathyamala, (eds.), 2006.

Satia, Jay, Dileep Mavalankar and Ramesh Bhat, 'Progress and Challenges of Health Sector: A Balance Sheet', Working Paper No. 99-10-08, October, 1999, IMM, Ahmedabad.

Sen, Binayak, 'A Suggested System for Undergraduate Medical Education', quoted in Doctors in Defence of Dr. Binayak Sen, *Indian Doctor in Jail*, Promilla & Co., New Delhi, 2008.

Sen, Gita, Aditi Iyer and Asha George, 'Structural Reform and Health Equity', *Economic and Political Weekly*, 6 April, 2002.

Shankar, Darshan, Agenda for Revitalisation of Indian Medical Heritage, Voluntary Health Association of India, New Delhi, 2001.

Shiva, Mira and Wishwas Rane, Banned and Bannable Drugs, Voluntary Health Association of India, New Delhi, 2004.

Sinha, Amarjeet, 'In Defence of the National Rural Health Mission', *Economic and Political Weekly*, 4 April, 2009

Voluntary Health Association of India, Report of the Independent Commission on Health, New Delhi, 1997.

World Trade Organisation, General Agreement on Trade in Services, 1995.

World Bank, 'World Development Report: Making Services Work for Poor People', 2004.

Notes

1. The NHFS-3 (data from 0–4 years back) finds an Infant Mortality Rate of 57. This implies that 57 children out of 1000 die before reaching the age of one year. The under-5 Child Mortality Rate is 74. Despite an improvement in position from what was reported by NHFS-2, these levels of IMR are disturbing and are higher than the target set in the Millennium Development Goals. The Maternal Mortality Rate is over 300 out of 100,000 deliveries and continues to be unacceptably high (JSA, 2009).
2. As per NHFS-3, full vaccine coverage in the last five years is 44%.
3. Around 3.7 lakh deaths from TB every year — the highest in the world.
4. Continuing high level of around 2 million cases annually of which nearly half are of Falciparum category (JSA, 2009).
5. Estimated to be at 31 lakh, the second highest in the world (JSA, 2009).
6. Nearly 6 lakh children die each year, which is easily preventable (JSA, 2009).
7. Rural Health Statistics of India, 2007.
8. As per a recent survey, 40% people could not seek treatment for ailments considered serious due to financial reasons (JSA, 2009).

Index